Praise for The Conscious

"These girls are the real deal. Their passionate approach to health, wellness, and weight loss is inspiring. They are both foodies who love to eat and detectives who will help you figure out what works on you. Plus, their recipes are fantastic—easy and delicious. Jo and Jules get it. The Conscious Cleanse is a program I highly recommend for anyone who wants to both feel and look better."

—Bobbi Brown, founder and chief creative officer, Bobbi Brown Cosmetics; beauty editor, *TODAY*

"The landscape of health has changed, and as we try to navigate conditions impacting our families today—diabetes, allergies, asthma, obesity and cancer—*The Conscious Cleanse* offers a practical and easy way to get started, offering a road map to health. Diet is like religion, it's not one size fits all, but this smart and practical guide offers ways to eliminate inflammatory triggers like allergens and empty calories, and offers shopping lists, recipes, and insight, making it a great resource for those wanting to get on the road to better health."

—Robyn O'Brien, dubbed "Food's Erin Brockovich" by *The New York Times*; author, *The Unhealthy Truth: How Our Food Is Making Us Sick and What We Can Do About It*; founder, AllergyKids Foundation; TEDx speaker

"I've witnessed firsthand how symptoms disappear and fast fat loss happens when people remove common food sensitivities. *The Conscious Cleanse* provides an easy-to-follow, effective, and fun strategy that helps you burn fat, ditch those nasty toxins, feel your sexiest, and turn back the clock 10 years. It asks for just 14 days, but when you see the results you'll stick with it forever."

—J. J. Virgin, CNS, CHFS; celebrity nutrition and fitness expert; host, Discovery Health's *Transformation Diaries*; co-star, TLC's *Freaky Eaters*; author, *Six Weeks to Sleeveless and Sexy* and *The Virgin Diet* (jjvirgin.com)

"*The Conscious Cleanse* is a call to action for all who are sick and tired of being sick and tired! Be ready to dig in the dirt to grow into the person you yearn to become. May your journey into vital health be an exquisite discovery and a walk in beauty."

—Ana T. Forrest, creatrix, Forrest Yoga; author, *Fierce Medicine;* ferocious autodidact

"Way more than just a fleeting detox program, *The Conscious Cleanse* took me on a modern-day journey into an intentional, awakened lifestyle. If you have ever felt alone in your quest for health, Jo and Jules hold your hand every step of the way, cheering you on with mouthwatering recipes, ace wellness tips, and positive encouragement. If you are ready to be fully alive, get with the Conscious Cleanse!"

—Amy Ippoliti, yoga instructor; founder, 90 Minutes to Change the World™

the conscious cleanse

Lose Weight, Heal Your Body, and Transform Your Life in 14 Days

Jo Schaalman and Julie Peláez
with Josh Dinar

ALPHA

A member of Penguin Group (USA) Inc.

ALPHA BOOKS

Published by Penguin Group (USA) Inc.

Penguin Group (USA) Inc., 375 Hudson Street, New York, New York 10014, USA • Penguin Group (Canada), 90 Eglinton Avenue East, Suite 700, Toronto, Ontario M4P 2Y3, Canada (a division of Pearson Penguin Canada Inc.) • Penguin Books Ltd., 80 Strand, London WC2R ORL, England • Penguin Ireland, 25 St. Stephen's Green, Dublin 2, Ireland (a division of Penguin Books Ltd.) • Penguin Group (Australia), 250 Camberwell Road, Camberwell, Victoria 3124, Australia (a division of Pearson Australia Group Pty. Ltd.) • Penguin Books India Pvt. Ltd., 11 Community Centre, Panchsheel Park, New Delhi—110 017, India • Penguin Group (NZ), 67 Apollo Drive, Rosedale, North Shore, Auckland 1311, New Zealand (a division of Pearson New Zealand Ltd.) • Penguin Books (South Africa) (Pty.) Ltd., 24 Sturdee Avenue, Rosebank, Johannesburg 2196, South Africa • Penguin Books Ltd., Registered Offices: 80 Strand, London WC2R ORL, England

International Standard Book Number: 978-1-61564-219-9
Library of Congress Catalog Card Number: 2012941774

14   8 7 6 5 4

Interpretation of the printing code: The rightmost number of the first series of numbers is the year of the book's printing; the rightmost number of the second series of numbers is the number of the book's printing. For example, a printing code of 12-1 shows that the first printing occurred in 2012.

Printed in the United States of America

Note: This publication contains the opinions and ideas of its authors. It is intended to provide helpful and informative material on the subject matter covered. It is sold with the understanding that the authors and publisher are not engaged in rendering professional services in the book. If the reader requires personal assistance or advice, a competent professional should be consulted.

The authors and publisher specifically disclaim any responsibility for any liability, loss, or risk, personal or otherwise, which is incurred as a consequence, directly or indirectly, of the use and application of any of the contents of this book.

Trademarks: All terms mentioned in this book that are known to be or are suspected of being trademarks or service marks have been appropriately capitalized. Alpha Books and Penguin Group (USA) Inc. cannot attest to the accuracy of this information. Use of a term in this book should not be regarded as affecting the validity of any trademark or service mark.

Most Alpha books are available at special quantity discounts for bulk purchases for sales promotions, premiums, fund-raising, or educational use. Special books, or book excerpts, can also be created to fit specific needs. For details, write: Special Markets, Alpha Books, 375 Hudson Street, New York, NY 10014.

Contents

Foreword

When you imagine a "cleanse," what do you think of? A fad or crash diet where you subsist on liquids alone? Spending hundreds of dollars on specialty foods you don't even like? Suffering or feeling on edge—somewhere between passing out and sprinting to the nearest doughnut shop? Or even worse, waking up a week later to realize you've somehow gained back the 10 pounds you lost?

That kind of "crash cleansing" is not what this book is about. A *conscious* cleanse is a much gentler, holistic process that teaches you how to pay attention to your body and its sensitivities. The end result may be weight loss, but more importantly, it will be a renewed sense of energy, satisfaction, and self-love.

Jules and Jo, the founders of the Conscious Cleanse, are an "odd couple" of health innovators with entirely different nutrition histories. Their firsthand experience proves that no one way of eating or cleansing works for everyone. That's the principle behind their exceptional 2-week program: a cleanse that can benefit and adapt to anyone, at any level of health, fitness, or happiness.

Increasingly, we live in a world where people are disconnected from their bodies. Whether we suffer from illnesses related to the standard American diet (SAD); deprive our bodies in an endless pursuit to be thin; or manipulate our bodies with aggressive, soul-crushing workouts, most of us share the same ailment: a complete and total disregard for the subtle, critical information our body provides on a daily basis. It's time to start trusting our bodies to know what's best for us, to stop ignoring the many signs and signals that can lead us to better health.

A conscious cleanse is not a diet. There is no calorie restriction, suffering, or starvation. Studies have shown that nearly 95 percent of people who "diet" gain back the weight within a year. This is about subtle shifts—in your awareness, in your taste buds, in your overall consciousness. An effective cleanse helps you uncover the power of your body's knowledge and discover what foods do or do not work for you. First and foremost, *The Conscious Cleanse* is an invitation to step back, to give yourself the gift of time, and to be attentive to the ways in which your habits may be preventing you from living your best life.

If you already lead a healthy lifestyle and think you feel great, consider this: most people don't realize how bad they feel until they start feeling better. Most of us have gotten so used to being fatigued, bloated, depressed, or plagued with illnesses like allergies or digestive problems that we consider those ailments normal. But what if you had the chance to feel extraordinary— to not only know that you live a healthy lifestyle, but to actually reap the benefits?

Having devoted my life to the study of health and wellness, I find the work of nutrition leaders like Jo and Jules a constant source of inspiration. They are the guides lighting our way out of the tunnel, sharing their experiences to help the rest of us achieve greater health and happiness. Taking back our bodies is not a complicated process, but it's not something we can achieve instantly. It's only through intentional thought, planning, and action that we can begin to recognize the obstacles that conspire against our health. But with the support of health leaders like Jo and Jules, whose personal battles have led them to contribute to the greater good, we can all learn to give ourselves the gift of health and create a ripple effect that, in turn, shares this gift with the rest of the world.

Joshua Rosenthal, MScEd

Joshua Rosenthal, MScED, is the founder and director of the Institute for Integrative Nutrition. He has worked in the nutrition field for more than 25 years, teaching at the school alongside health leaders such as Andrew Weil, Deepak Chopra, and Barry Sears. At Integrative Nutrition, students are trained as Health Coaches, receiving the holistic nutrition education necessary for them go out into the world and help others improve their health and happiness.

Introduction

Food is our common ground, a universal experience.

—James Beard

Are you ready to transform your life? You're about to embark on an amazing journey of self-discovery and awareness, one that will produce profound and lasting results. And one that's grounded equally in science and good, old-fashioned common sense.

If there's anything we've learned in the years we've been guiding participants through the Conscious Cleanse, it's that nothing helps make sense of a complex relationship with food like simplification. So we're going to simplify. There's no greater gift you can give yourself than a fresh start. At the other end of this program, you'll be well on your way to your ideal weight, you'll feel refreshed and clear-headed, and, most importantly, you'll better understand how your body responds to the things you put in it.

So in a nutshell, here's the program:

Step 1: Commit. Give yourself the gift of 14 days. And while you're here, really throw yourself into the process. Try things, even if they seem silly to you. Keep a journal. Taste kale. Make time for a 2-hour dinner on a Wednesday night. (Yes, you read that right!) It's all do-able, we promise. Tell yourself, *This is an experiment I'm committed to. I'm going to step out of my comfort zone for the next two weeks.* You'll be amazed at what suddenly seems possible when you start breaking old habits.

Step 2: Slow down. We know you probably have a very busy life. But here's what we've learned from the participants in our programs over the years: you don't *find* time; you *make* it. As a part of your 14-day experiment, put your multitasking aside temporarily. Take a breath. Take another. Focus on the task at hand. Don't rush through. During the Conscious Cleanse, we practice the ever-elusive art of *savoring*. If you feel yourself begin to hurry during the program, slow yourself down, even if only for a moment. Savoring food is a metaphor for savoring time. And when you savor time, you savor your life.

Step 3: Prepare. We repeat: you don't *find* time; you *make* it. Having a plan for tomorrow allows you to live in the moment today. Practically speaking, we suggest you read Part 1 of this book before beginning your official cleanse. Spontaneity may be the spice of life, but it's not ideal for managing your diet. So by all means, go dancing on a whim, but if you know you want to eat specific foods during your meals and snacks tomorrow, you should probably be sure you have what you need in the house.

Read the chapters on preparing to cleanse, explore the recipes and shopping list at the back of the book, and plan your meals. Being prepared means you won't get caught hungry and start sliding into forage mode. Being prepared means you know brown rice takes 45 minutes to cook. Being prepared means you know how you're going to deal with your friend's birthday dinner at a restaurant before the first breadbasket arrives at the table. Preparedness trumps willpower every day of the week (and twice on purification weekends).

Step 4: Eat. And eat consciously. No starving yourself! Aside from being a miserable experience, it doesn't work. In Part 1, we discuss what you'll leave off your plate during the program so you can understand the theory behind the Conscious Cleanse. When we have that out of the way, we do an about-face from that focus. Where the mind goes, the energy flows, so instead of concentrating on what *not* to eat, we focus on what you *get to* eat as you step into Part 2 and begin your cleanse.

In fact, you are going to learn a whole new appreciation for eating. Your body goes into a defense mode when it senses it's being deprived. So for starters, don't deprive yourself. For each of the 14 days, we offer sample meal plans, tips for sticking with the program, and small inspirations and "action items." We know eating is so rarely just about food, so we pay attention to both the body and the mind as we move through the process.

The Conscious Cleanse is about true nourishment. You can have everything you want—an ideal weight; a life free of aches, pains, and illness; boundless energy; and mental clarity—simply by giving your body what it truly wants.

Step 5: Learn from your experience. Trust us, if you stick with the Conscious Cleanse, you're going to feel good at the end of it. In Part 3, we guide you through a gentle reintroduction of foods, using your "clean slate" as an opportunity to gain even more insight into your body's reactions—both physically and emotionally—to food.

Going forward, you'll be making more informed decisions and have a closer connection to the reasons why you're eating. You'll have gained a whole new perspective on your relationship to food—a perspective you'll be able to draw on and come back to for the rest of your life. At its core, the Conscious Cleanse is about empowerment. Not gaining new power, necessarily, but tapping into a power you already have inside of you. If you're open to it, if you pay attention to it and nurture it, that power can guide you toward true vibrancy, and suddenly everything will seem possible.

You Are Not Alone: A Brief History of the Conscious Cleanse

No two people are the same. Our bodies are intricate pulses of energy, each one unique in so many ways. Too New Age-y? Maybe, but it's true that you're the only one who knows what it's like to be you. The way you feel, the way you think, and the way you perceive the world are yours alone.

Yet you're not alone. We have our separate experiences and our separate bodies in common. That's the beauty of being human, and it's the basis for the Conscious Cleanse. The 14-day journey you're about to embark upon is a guide to designing your own path to vibrant health. There is no one-size-fits-all solution, but we can share in the ride.

We are perfect examples of this. We came together from opposite sides of the health spectrum. Jules, for example, has been blessed with relatively exceptional health. Her motivation to develop a program came from a lifetime of being in tune with her body, from a fervent drive to explore the relationship between food and the body, and a personal quest for optimal health. Over the years, Jules has been inspired by, and learned from, those she's met who have overcome significant ailments, those she's seen improve their lives through their food choices. Jules herself, though, is one of the lucky ones—her own motivation comes from a desire to maintain (rather than *attain*) vibrancy in her life.

Jo, on the other hand, was born with such severe allergies that her finger swelled if it so much as touched a tomato. She could not eat food cooked in plastic without getting a rash. Gluten, dairy, eggs, yeast, avocados, mangoes, lentils, apples, pears, grapes, cherries—you name it, and chances are it caused some kind of allergic reaction, often severe. Jo couldn't tolerate chemicals or fragrances, so her mother had to clean with vinegar and baking soda. She had to avoid pesticides, carpeting, and pets. Her seasonal allergies made the simple act of breathing a labored chore. She spent most of her childhood spring seasons hunched over a sink of steaming water to help ease her severe asthma.

Doctors told her mother Jo was an anomaly—that it's highly uncommon for someone to be so reactive to food and environment. Looking back, Jo thinks of her younger self as a canary in a coal mine.

Jo credits her mother, who walked out of countless doctors' offices, convinced there was a solution beyond the medicated breathing machine and high-dose prescriptions. Jo and her mother eventually found Theron Randolph, a forward-thinking doctor, recognized as the "father" of environmental medicine and the field of clinical ecology, who believed that most physical and mental diseases could be attributed to food and environmental toxins. He devised for Jo a natural plan that began with a rotation diet, where she ate only one type of food per day. Jo's new diet completely eliminated the need for medication. She got healthier, and she thrived.

Seventeen years later, Jo was a hard-working competitive diver and straight A college grad preparing to attend medical school. Before buckling down to start her life as a doctor, Jo took a summer job leading a cross-country bicycle trip for teenagers, and the course of her life once again took a dramatic turn.

On July 26, 2004, on a desert highway outside of Tuba City, Arizona, Jo was hit by a truck travelling 70 miles per hour. She was thrown from her bicycle and suffered severe spinal fractures and other serious injuries. Once again Jo found herself confronted by doctors who told her she would be "disabled" for the rest of her life, that she would have to learn to cope with severe chronic pain. She couldn't sit, walk, or stand, much less run, bike, or swim, and her dreams of medical school were put on hold indefinitely.

Athlete, overachiever, hard worker, aspiring doctor—every way she'd defined herself—in an instant, was gone. She gained 25 pounds on her 5 foot 1 frame. She was depressed and hopeless, without direction. Who would she be? What kind of life could she live? Who would love her?

Jo spent the next 2 years in and out of doctor's offices.

She took on her healing as she'd taken on the rest of her life: work harder and push through the pain. She saw a dozen specialists a week: massage therapists, acupuncturists, physical therapists, anyone who might give her hope. The one thing she didn't do, however, was slow down, listen to her body, or tap into her innate wisdom.

Jo spent years "trying harder" to heal. She struggled and pushed against herself. She took countless pills and injections to numb the pain, but her body's old sensitivities couldn't tolerate the medication, and she didn't want to live in a drugged fog that left her apathetic and disconnected from the world and herself. So she summoned the wisdom of her mother, who knew there was a different way, and she refused to sacrifice optimal health for symptom masking. And that's when her true healing began.

Jo took on yoga as a means to manage the physical pain. She worked with another forward-thinking healer, Ana Forrest, to find what her physical, emotional, and spiritual body needed. She experimented with various diets and programs. The process was ripe with trial and error, and she continued to obsess over her weight. She spent time trying strict programs and experimenting with extreme cleanses. Nothing worked. She read countless books on the latest and greatest ways to lose weight. She wanted her pain to go away, but she was at odds with her body and was approaching her health from a weight-loss perspective first. Being overweight, in many ways, she thought, made her more miserable than the constant physical pain.

When the two of us met, we found we shared a love and a fascination with the healing powers of food. Drawing from each other's experiences helped us assemble the pieces of our own puzzles. Jules is tall; Jo is short. Jules is brunette; Jo is blond. Jules is long and lean; Jo is muscular. Jules doesn't eat meat; Jo does. In many ways we look like the odd couple.

But even in our wild differences, there are deep commonalities. We found healing and vibrant health using similar overarching principles, but we individualized our approach for our own bodies, our own unique chemical makeups. From our partnership, we learned there's no one-size-fits-all blueprint to optimal health. We learned that you start from a common ground, and you customize from there to suit your needs. You will see this acknowledgment of diversity utilized throughout the Conscious Cleanse.

What happened for Jo as we continued to develop the Conscious Cleanse was nothing short of revelatory. Every single thing she ate came with the question, "How will this make me feel?" She combined her childhood doctor's method of isolating foods with updated academic and clinical knowledge, listened to her body, and worked to understand what foods caused greater levels of inflammation and what caused pain. She worked closely with Jules, who constantly challenged and inspired her to think about her health and diet in new ways. More greens, less meat. Eliminate allergens completely. With the support of her many teachers, Jo became fierce with her healing.

Eventually, Jo's daily pain levels went from a 7 to a 3. She dropped 15 pounds almost immediately. Her thyroid, which had been nearly nonfunctional, kicked in. Her recovery took quantum leaps, and one day she realized she actually felt better, in many ways, than she had before the accident. In the face of these results, we knew we'd struck on something.

And that *something* is the basis of the book you're holding in your hands—a program we developed through our various workshops and the ever-expanding community of Conscious Cleansers who've found their own version of optimal health. The Conscious Cleanse is built on what we've learned for ourselves and from others: that from flexibility and compassion comes sustainability; that from community and sharing comes individual power.

Are you ready? Because you're about to prove just how powerful you are.

Treat the Symptoms: A Home Repair Analogy

Start your journey with a bold statement:

>   I don't want another diet.

If you're here to lose weight, chances are you've lost it before. And gained it. And lost it. And gained it. Why is that such a common phenomenon?

Indulge us an analogy: one day, you notice a crack in the wall of your house. You resolve to fix it. You set aside a Saturday morning, head to the hardware store, buy spackle and tape and sandpaper and a trowel, and you spend the next couple hours thoroughly repairing the crack. When you're done, you paint over it, matching it carefully to ensure the color blends. You stand back and admire your work. The wall is fixed, good as new.

But a couple months later, the crack is back, and it's longer and wider than it was before. You can fix it again, right? You've fixed it before. What are the chances it will hold this time?

Obviously, the crack is not the problem. It's the symptom. The symptom can be covered up over and over again, but that won't make the problem go away. The problem lies in the foundation. It may be more work to fix foundations, but here's the thing: when that work is done, its benefits are drastic and long lasting. The crack doesn't come back, but more than that, new cracks don't form; you've shored things up so your house is better equipped to withstand wind and rain and there's less strain on pipes and wires.

We think you get the point. Your extra weight, your lack of energy, your migraines, your aches and pains, your stress, your insomnia, your allergies and illnesses—these are but examples of possible cracks in the house that is your body.

During the 2 weeks of the Conscious Cleanse, we're going to help you get down into the basement, clear out the cobwebs, organize, declutter, and set the stage for true foundational change. And if you're currently symptom free, all the better! Cleaning up and performing maintenance is how you stay that way. You'll find that you already have most of the tools you need and the work is easier than you imagined.

So back to our bold statement: you don't want another diet. So many of us put the proverbial cart before the horse. We think that if we lose weight we'll feel better about ourselves, so we cut corners, engage in weird fasts, eat only cabbage and broth, or deprive ourselves in some other unsustainable way to accomplish that end. And we do feel better for a bit. But the spackle doesn't hold.

You don't want another diet. What you really want is a happy and symptom-free life. You want to feel like your best self. You want to feel in control. Once you've got all that, the rest—including your weight—just falls into place.

Consciousness begins with choice. In picking up this book, you've already made the choice to show up, to engage. Congratulations on taking that huge first step. We're so glad you're here.

How the Conscious Cleanse Differs

We created the Conscious Cleanse for ourselves first, while on our own quest for vibrant health, ideal body weight, and personal healing. As we share it with you, our goal is to help you design your own perfect diet. The Conscious Cleanse is like a base camp, a place you can return to repeatedly to catch your breath and recharge. But like any base camp, it's designed to encourage exploration beyond its borders.

Our goal is to help set you up for optimal health and vibrancy for the rest of your life, and we know that with that lofty goal, deprivation cannot be part of the equation. Like a marriage, a career, or any proud achievement, there are no shortcuts to success. The work must be done, but with the right mind-set, the work—as well as its outcomes—can be joyful.

Not Required: Willpower or Expensive Supplements

There's no doubt about it: cleansing is all the rage. We've got juice fasts and liquid diets coming out the yin yang. We're bombarded by companies trying to sell us expensive supplements (by the way, we discuss supplements in the "Preparing to Cleanse" chapter). But the fact of the matter is that you don't need to starve or heavily restrict yourself, and you don't need pills because you can get all the nutrients you need from actual food.

Most importantly, the Conscious Cleanse is not a "diet." It's not an all-or-nothing proposition. It's not about "just pushing through." It's meant to be accessible, to meet you where you are and to celebrate the fact that we are all individuals. The program is not calorie restricted. As with any habit changing, the cleanse takes your active and conscious participation, but it's not about suffering, either physically or emotionally.

During the 14 days of the program, we guide you through a gentle detoxification of your system and simultaneously help you design a sustainable way of eating catered specifically for you. At the end of the program, we guide you through a reintegration. You'll take all you've learned about yourself—trust us, it will be a lot!—and use it to help you draw a road map for maintaining your stunningly renewed sense of vibrancy.

Focus on Allergens and Participants' Unique Identities

For 2 weeks, you're going to flush your system and give it a chance to rest and recuperate. During that time, you keep the foods that can potentially tax your system—the allergens—off your plate.

Some of these foods—like tomatoes, oranges, and eggs—may seem counter-intuitive at first. But the fact of the matter is that statistics estimate up to 90 percent of Americans suffer from food intolerances or allergies, and most are undetected.

That bears repeating. A whopping 9 out of 10 people may have some form of food intolerance, and most of those people don't connect the food they're eating to the physical ailments they're experiencing: cramps, diarrhea or constipation, headaches, clogged sinuses, lethargy, aches and pains, and a number of much more serious conditions.

Many people with food allergies or sensitivities are actually "addicted" to the foods causing the problems. Crave cheese or dairy? Can't go a day without eggs? This information may be the key to unlocking the truth about what's causing you problems. The sneaky thing about allergens is that sometimes when you remove them from your diet, you actually feel worse initially. Think about alcohol. When you wake up after a night of overindulgence feeling foggy and sluggish, it's the bloody Mary that takes the edge off. Food allergies work just like this so-called "hair of the dog" effect.

By avoiding or limiting the possible culprit foods for a couple weeks, you give your digestive system a much-needed rest. During this time, your body flushes out built-up toxins, allowing you the opportunity to isolate different foods' effects on you and experience just how well your body can heal itself, given the chance.

It's that experience that will guide you to your own answers, to the development of your own perfect diet—a diet that helps eliminate toxins on an ongoing basis so you no longer carry around extra weight or suffer from countless medical conditions, big or small.

Design and Reintegration

It's from this clean slate that you can begin to cultivate a deeper understanding of yourself. That may sound hokey, but truly, you can't organize your basement until you've cleaned it out, removed the trash, and taken inventory. If you pay attention during the 2 weeks of the Conscious Cleanse, take the time to tune inward, and listen to your body—your own intuitive voice—you'll come out with answers that can inform countless decisions.

The Conscious Cleanse is based on just a handful of some very simple eating practices—ideas that have been around since the beginning of time. We're not offering any groundbreaking "diet" information here. We're simply helping uncover what you already know at a cellular and intuitive level.

At the end of the Conscious Cleanse, you won't want to return to your old habits. We guide you through a thoughtful and purposeful reintegration of foods so your sense of renewed vigor and natural weight stay with you.

Which leads us to a confession: the Conscious Cleanse is not really just a 2-week program. It was developed as a means to give you a clean slate, a fresh start, a blank canvas upon which you can design a "food lifestyle" of your very own. At the end of the program, you'll have developed a way of eating that supports your genetic blueprint and fits naturally into your daily life—one that delivers vibrant health, natural weight loss, and boundless energy, and one that's sustainable for a lifetime!

The Importance of Journaling

We'll reiterate throughout this book that food is never just about food. Think about it. How often do we really use our food as fuel? Why is it that we have to have a "relationship" with food? It will come as no surprise that food creates emotional responses within us, and getting a hold of your diet means making the effort to get in touch with that. One of the most powerful things you can do to take charge of what goes in your mouth is to take charge of what's in your head.

Maybe that's a little counterintuitive, but the fact of the matter is that it's surprisingly easy to go about our days without considering the motives for our actions, especially the ones that, on the surface, seem the simplest, like eating. Much of the Conscious Cleanse is about breaking that mold, becoming *present* for even the seemingly mundane aspects of our lives. When you're present, you can't help but have an appreciation for your everyday life. Suddenly even the mundane begins to take on new shape, and the world begins to seem full of possibilities. This is the power of exploring your thoughts, and we're going to challenge you to do it carefully throughout this book via journaling.

We can't overstate just how crucial a component journaling is to your 2-week commitment. Make this part of your experiment, part of your journey, and pay attention to the empowerment that comes from archiving your thoughts and exploring your motivations. This commitment alone has the power to transform your life.

Start today. Notice any resistance you have to the idea right now, and consider that even more of a reason to find yourself a blank notebook or a journal. Grab a pen and allow yourself to simply start writing what comes to mind, even if you end up writing "I think journal writing is stupid and doesn't work for me." Write uncensored for just 5 minutes today.

We discuss more on journal writing in Day 1 of the program, and throughout the 2 weeks, we provide journal prompts and things to consider to help get you journaling each day.

What to Expect from the Conscious Cleanse

In the coming chapters, we offer you an overview of the Conscious Cleanse and prepare you to begin your 14-day program. At this point, we've heard the gamut of emotions from our participants—from dread to excitement, from fear and anxiousness to optimistic hope. Any and all of these are natural responses to the unknown, indicators that you're stepping out of your comfort zone, which is the only place real transformation happens. So whatever you're feeling, don't ignore it, and don't sweat it. Be present. Pay attention to what-ever comes up for you, and observe how it changes as you move forward.

There's often a desire—especially from those who have tried a cleanse before—to set expectations, to be mentally prepared for a physical challenge.

Will I be tired? Will I have energy? Will I get headaches? Will my sleep be affected? Will I have to alter my exercise routine? Will I have cravings? And so on. The answer to all these questions is a resounding *maybe*.

We've said it before and we'll say it again: this is an individualized process. Each of our bodies reacts differently to change, based on any number of factors. If we can make one overarching statement, it's this: when you change your inputs, you should be prepared for different outputs. The changes may be very subtle, or they may be very dramatic. They may come in the form of increased energy and enhanced libido, or they may come in the form of nausea and headaches. Or more likely, they'll be a little of each.

Keep in mind as you start the program that your body is undergoing a detoxification and reprogramming, that it's withdrawing from what might be many years of certain inputs. We'll urge you to stay with it in that first week, to embrace whatever form your change rides in on, to listen, be conscious, and respond accordingly. The Conscious Cleanse, much unlike other cleanses, is not a pass-or-fail proposition. There is no wagon, so there's no wagon to fall off of. We welcome you to tailor, to tinker, to tweak and adjust as necessary. We offer hints and suggestions on a daily basis along the way.

Let's go back to our earlier analogy for a moment. Cleaning out the basement allows you to get to the foundation. But a cluttered basement doesn't become cluttered overnight. It takes years of storing things you don't really need, little by little. Clearing it out can be done in far less time than it took to junk it up—it just takes some dedicated attention to make a remarkable difference. The same is true in your body: trust the cleaning process, and relatively quickly, you'll notice things start to come into focus.

The Conscious Cleanse is designed to be gentle and accessible. Parts of it will certainly seem very easy. Some parts may seem challenging. Which parts are which? That's different for everyone.

During your 14 days, you should expect to step out of your comfort zone but not to be exceptionally uncomfortable. Stretch, but don't tear. Confront yourself, but never assault yourself. The program is 14 days, but today is just 1 day, and tomorrow is another. So don't rush ahead. Relish the journey. Most important, expect to surprise yourself.

With love and green veggies,
Jules and Jo

PS: Please visit consciouscleanse.com for special cleanse documents and downloads, additional recipes, and a fast-growing community of people taking their health to the level of vibrancy with the Conscious Cleanse.

Acknowledgments

From Jo and Jules: It's with heartfelt joy and appreciation that we thank Kate and Josh Dinar. If Kate hadn't roped Josh into taking the cleanse with her in August 2011, this book would not exist today. And to Josh—for seeing something in us, for believing in us and our program. We are forever grateful to you. Our amazing team of editors at Alpha—Lori, Christy, and Cate—made the sometimes-daunting task of completing this book a true joy. We thank you for your inspiring professionalism, good humor, patience, and incredible attention to detail. To all our cleanse participants—thank you for trusting us to lovingly guide and nurture your healing process and transformation. Without you, this program would not exist. And to Annie—the "Queen of Poop Talk," who taught us much of what we know about cleansing the colon—thank you for loving us unconditionally.

From Jo: Jules, you are the yin to my yang, the tall to my short. This book would never have been written without you. My dad, thank you being a dreamer, creator, and idealist. You've taught me how to pick myself up when I'm down, be resilient, and live with purpose. My mom, this book is an expression of my gratitude for you. Thank you for following your intuition, for being selfless, and for your unwavering tenacity. My grandparents, thank you for being my wise mentors, for teaching me what it means to live with real purpose and passion. My loving husband-to-be, Adam, thank you for your steadfast love, your support, and being king of the Vitamix during the highs and lows of this creative process. It's no coincidence that my life began to flow as soon as you came into it. Ana, thank you for believing I could heal and teaching me how to do it myself.

From Jules: My sweet friend, Jo, thank you for inviting me to be on this journey with you and for always bringing me back to Earth. Every "Ay ya ya" and "Oy!" has been a joy because of our true partnership. Enzo, my spreader of joy, thank you for loving every green smoothie I ever conjure up. I will forever cherish our first actual conversation containing the words "cilantro, kale, and yum." And Rocco, the original Conscious Cleanse baby, thank you for peacefully sitting beside me as I wrote and for being my constant reminder of the Great Mystery. And Digger, you are my rock—thank you for showing me the way and loving me unconditionally. I love you.

From Josh: My "angels," Jo and Jules, your work is nothing short of inspiring. You made every second of this project a pleasure, and it's my deepest honor to be a part of it. I look forward to the wide-open frontier in front of us. Mason, who loves any food he's ever tried except quinoa and pancakes, and Levi, who can drink a green smoothie with his whole face—thank you for giving me the two greatest gifts a person can have in his life: laughter and awe. And Katie, I have no idea how a chucklehead like me ends up with the most patient, loyal, loving, gorgeous soul that exists, but I ain't complaining. You're my reason why.

Part 1

Becoming Food Conscious

Why Cleanse?

Food is an important part of a balanced diet.

—Fran Lebowitz

Start where you are. The guidance you get from this book is no more profound than that. *Start where you are.* Sounds pretty obvious, doesn't it? But how often do we truly give ourselves that gift? How often do we stop and tell ourselves that wherever we're headed, *this* is where we start? It means being willing to forgive the past. It means controlling the urge to race ahead.

Sometimes the simplest truths are the most slippery. In so many ways, the Conscious Cleanse is about learning what you already know—following intuition and going with your gut. To that end, we begin with a short self-evaluation, the Conscious Wellness Evaluation, the first of many times during the Conscious Cleanse you stop and take a moment to listen to yourself. As with the entire program, there are no wrong answers—no shame, no judgment. The Conscious Wellness Evaluation serves as your baseline. We ask you to come back to it throughout the program, and especially at the end, to examine your progress and help gauge the gains you've made in your overall well-being by eating consciously.

Then, throughout the rest of this chapter we explore the reasons for cleansing in some more depth, discuss the impact of "food demons" on your system, get down and dirty with some "poop talk," and take a look at some distractions—the things that tend to get between you and your optimal health.

The Conscious Wellness Evaluation

Before you begin making any dietary changes, please take 5 minutes to fill out this evaluation as honestly and openly as possible. If you're feeling extra adventurous, take a picture of yourself, too! It'll be nice to have a "before" shot.

On a scale of 1 to 10, with 10 being "Amazing!" rate yourself on how you feel about the following areas of your health/life.

	Day 1	Day 7	Day 14
Allergies			
Appetite			
Body aches and pains			
Bowel movements			
Cravings			
Energy			
Hair			
Hormonal cycles			
Immune system			
Memory			
Mental clarity			
Mood			
Outlook on life			
Skin condition			
Sleep			
Stress level			

You revisit this form on Day 7 and again on Day 14.

Reducing the Impact of Toxins

Toxins are everywhere. It's a fact of living in the modern, convenient world. We're regularly exposed to environmental pollutants, pesticides, herbicides, processed food, chemical preservatives, genetically modified food, and animal products filled with antibiotics and growth hormones.

As a culture, we've become accustomed to eating bread, milk, pasta, cheese, processed snack foods, soda, and sugary treats on a daily basis. The quality of our food choices has been hijacked by convenience, and as a result, we're ingesting more gluten, sugar, and genetically modified corn than ever before. More often than not, we don't even know when we're eating these things. According to Dr. John Douillard, director of the LifeSpa Ayurvedic Center, even our field-grown *organic* food contains trace amounts of mercury from the falling rain.

When you start to look, it seems like trace amounts of something are in just about everything. It makes sense that over the years, all those trace amounts add up. As a result, your body—specifically your detoxification organs like your liver and kidneys—become overloaded. Your system grows clogged, and a clogged system can't function at full capacity. Is it any wonder you don't feel like your best self?

Allergies Galore

Some estimates suggest up to 90 percent of Americans suffer from allergies, and most of those go undetected.

The good news is that your body is designed to filter toxins from your environment. While it would be a silly and lost cause to try to avoid all toxins on a day-to-day basis, it *is* possible, and even relatively easy, to greatly reduce your exposure, giving your body a much-needed rest.

In our programs, we sometimes ask participants to describe the way they take care of their cars. Tire rotations, oil changes, clean filters, new sparkplugs—you perform routine maintenance on your automobile like clockwork because you know (or are told by your mechanic) that these seemingly simple things will keep it running longer and more efficiently.

What if you let your car go an extra 1,000 miles before changing the oil? Probably not the end of the world, right? It would probably drive the same. How about 5,000 miles or 10,000 or even 40,000? At what point does the car start to make weird noises? When does the acceleration start getting sluggish? When does the intermittent sputtering kick in? And how long before you're stranded on the side of the road?

Well, your body is a machine, too. And you can think of the Conscious Cleanse as an oil and filter change for that machine—a small but imperative diversion that can keep you running smoothly and extend the length and quality of your life.

The Medical and Health Benefits of the Conscious Cleanse

The Conscious Cleanse is based in some very straightforward, relatively uncontroversial science. The bottom line is that the food that's most convenient, most inexpensive, and most readily available to us is making us sick.

But there is good news: in recent years, the pendulum has begun to swing back the other way. Labels and certifications like the USDA Organic certification have made knowing what we're putting in our bodies much simpler, and an increase in demand for healthier food has made it easier to choose a dietary lifestyle that supports—rather than hinders—health.

The Energy of Digestion

Mark Twain, infamous lover of decadent food, said, "Part of the secret of success in life is to eat what you like and let the food fight it out inside." Of course, Twain was joking, but part of what makes a joke funny is that we "get it."

Put aside for a moment the fact that Twain lived in the 1800s, when organic food was just called food; when animals, whose diet also consisted of food, were raised in pastures; and when food wasn't responsible for public epidemics of diabetes and obesity. Put aside the new dangers that exist today, and just think about some words to describe the way you feel after a big, rich, decadent meal—a meal at which you'd say you'd "overeaten." We're guessing the words you come up with don't include *energetic* or *vibrant*.

That sluggish, bloated, fatigued feeling you're likely conjuring? The gas? The heartburn? That, as Twain quipped, is "the food fighting it out inside." This isn't to say a little indulgence from time to time isn't a valid part of the human experience; it's simply to illustrate that it takes a tremendous amount of energy to digest food.

In fact, over the course of an average person's lifetime, about 80 percent of the body's energy goes toward digestion. Think about that for a minute. Of all the energy you consume, only 20 percent is available to bodily functions, including your immune system, your cardiovascular system, your liver, your kidneys, and your brain. It's a simple, intuitive formula: the more you eat (and especially the more highly processed or complex foods), the harder your body has to work to digest, and the less energy is available to your body's other tasks.

Now imagine if you could improve that efficiency. Every percentage point of energy you free up goes toward the maintenance and healing of your body. You're better able to fight infection, you think more clearly, you have less inflammation, you experience fewer aches and pains, you recover more quickly from physical exertion, and you have more vigor.

The Toll of Toxins

Now add back in the "toxin factor"—the additional strain put on your system by the need to deal with the elimination of chemicals—and suddenly the growing diet-related health concerns in this country make a whole lot of sense. It's a simple and intuitive formula: if you consume fewer toxins by eating

"cleaner" food, you'll reduce the energy your body requires to d
elimination. The Conscious Cleanse is designed to give your live
and other detoxification organs a much-needed rest. As in our car
the less taxed these organs are, the more efficiently they'll function—and the
longer they'll last.

During the Conscious Cleanse, you'll be naturally eating as close to a toxin-free diet as possible, giving your body a chance to rest and repair at a cellular level. There's a "snowball effect" to this kind of system cleansing: your body has more energy to repair itself and ultimately there's less to repair. Many of our participants describe experiencing a "boundless energy" as the cleanse progresses; they feel as if their bodies are no longer racing to keep up. And magically, symptoms begin to disappear.

Think about it: more energy, less illness. Suddenly, you're able to focus more clearly, to be *present* in your life. The effects of the cleanse, as we've already suggested, go far beyond just weight loss, offering a sense of true *vitality*.

Reassessing Standards

The standard American diet has an unfortunate but apt acronym: *SAD*. In the United States, the typical diet is laden with dairy, gluten, yeast, sugar, corn, animal and saturated fats, simple carbohydrates, caffeine, and alcohol, not to mention chemicals and preservatives. Conversely, the SAD is sorely lacking in fiber and nutrient-dense, plant-based foods.

There's little argument against the claims that this "standard" diet has created major health problems in this country. Historically high rates of obesity, diabetes, heart disease, cancer, high blood pressure, and high cholesterol have become the status quo, as has the tendency to treat these "symptoms" with pills. But the fact is that countries where the dietary norm is opposite of ours have markedly lower levels of these ailments.

Aside from contributing to significant health problems, the SAD serves to slow the digestive system, resulting in a tarlike buildup on the intestinal walls. After many years of accumulation, a mucus lining is created, and this lining actually inhibits the absorption of essential vitamins, minerals, and nutrients from our food.

We've also become a society addicted to convenience. Our food is ready and waiting for us wherever we are and whenever we want it—and we don't have time for it to be any other way. The cost of that convenience is not knowing whether the food we're eating is harmful to us or not. And when it turns out that it is, we're sold on more quick fixes—a pill for every symptom.

Overprescribed Cholesterol Drugs

More than 200 million prescriptions for cholesterol-reducing drugs are written every year in the United States. Seems strange, considering cholesterol often can be lowered with a healthy diet. Clinical nutrition researcher Neal Barnard, MD, founder and president of the Physicians Committee for Responsible Medicine, suggests a "month-long experiment" to his patients. Remove all animal products and increase vegetables, fruits, whole grains, and beans and see what happens.

During the Conscious Cleanse, we're going to steer you clear of the possible "culprit" foods, most of which have become staples of the SAD. This is a crucial piece of your experiment, whether or not you think these foods are actually causing you problems. In fact, most of our participants believe that some of the things we suggest keeping off the plate for these 2 weeks aren't problems for them. And that's okay! In fact, that's a major part of the opportunity you're giving yourself. You may be surprised by what you learn!

Conscious Success Story: Lowering Cholesterol

Ben, a 58-year-old attorney, travels a lot for work. One morning at a hotel breakfast, he ordered grapefruit juice. One of his colleagues, upon hearing his request, exclaimed, "You know you can't drink that on your cholesterol medication, right?" When Ben told his colleague he wasn't on any medication, the whole table was shocked. Ben was the only one of the group not on a cholesterol drug. He was surprised that his peers took their own medications in such stride, that high cholesterol was so standard among them it could be assumed everyone was on something for it.

A few months later, Ben's doctor informed him that he, like his fellow attorneys at that breakfast, also had high cholesterol. The doctor suggested a medication to control it. Ben considered himself a relatively healthy person, though, and asked the doctor to give him 6 months to try to bring his cholesterol down naturally.

After participating in the Conscious Cleanse, Ben recognized that what he'd considered a "heart-healthy" diet actually had high levels of sugar hidden in it. His daily oatmeal, juice, condiments, and sauces were slowly creating a problem for him. He kept these things out of his diet for several months after the cleanse and continued to consume more veggies in the form of a morning smoothie. When he returned for his follow-up, he learned his cholesterol had dropped by more than 75 points, astounding his doctor.

The Mental Reboot

The last reason we cleanse, and maybe the least obvious, is so we can slow down, tune in, and hit the reboot button. Most of us are living very full, very fast-paced daily lives. Think of the benefits of a long and relaxing beach vacation. How much more productive are you upon your return? How much easier is it to deal with daily stresses?

A healthy cleanse, like a vacation, forces you to naturally slow down. You take time to shop and prepare your food. You pay attention to eating again, savoring new flavors and textures. Even a small act, like slicing a cucumber, if you pay attention to it, will give you a deeper connection to your food and awaken your senses. The food you eat feeds your cells, your blood, your tissues, and your bones. So when you connect to that food, you're connecting more deeply to yourself. You are, in this sense, quite literally what you eat.

Slowing Down

Every time I do this cleanse I'm amazed how it reminds me to prep good food, eat my food more slowly, and actually slow down in all aspects of my life.

—Jules K., a frequent Conscious Cleanser

Slowing down causes a ripple effect. As you begin to examine your food choices, you naturally start to look at your relationships, your finances, your work, your outlook on life, your dreams, etc. So if you decided to do this program with the goal of losing weight, rest assured, you will get results. But what you may not realize is that weight loss is just scratching the surface. The weight will come off naturally, and will naturally stay off, as you dig deeper, as you begin to explore the endless possibilities of a vibrant and conscious existence.

Sounds promising, doesn't it?

Let's get started on cleaning up your diet. A conscious new you is waiting!

In the Bathroom ...

One of the first questions we ask our participants is, "How's your stool?" While you might not want to try it at a dinner party, in the right situation it can be a highly effective icebreaker. The response, after the initial shock wears off, is usually the same across the board: uncomfortable giggles, averted eyes, and a sheepish, hesitant version of, "It's fine, I guess."

Your bowel movements can tell you a lot about your health. They can tell you if you're digesting your food properly and in a timely manner. They can alert you to possible allergies, malabsorption, and even chronic disease and illness. But first you have to be going!

Our Diet Is Killing Us

According to the American Cancer Society, colorectal cancer is the third most commonly diagnosed cancer and the third leading cause of cancer death in both men and women in the United States. Need another reason to cleanse the colon?

Most Americans consider it "normal" to miss a day here and there. Or they believe they're "regular" because they go once a day, even though that once a day consists of some serious bearing down for 20 minutes. Many people suffer from diarrhea or have mucus in their stool. These symptoms, along with gas and bloating, are signs of an unhealthy colon. Some experts even go as far as saying that if you're not consistently eliminating within an hour of waking, you're constipated! The longer waste sits in your body, the more you face the nasty risk of those toxins being reabsorbed and flushed into your bloodstream. Yuck!

Unhealthy stool is a symptom, a warning sign—consider it the "Check Oil" light on your dashboard. But enough of the doom and gloom. Let's talk about what a *healthy* elimination looks like.

Signs of healthy colon function include these:

- Your stool is soft and easy to pass.
- It's about a foot long, and breaks apart when you flush.
- It floats and is relatively odor free.
- You eliminate two or three times per day, ideally within an hour of waking up and after every meal.
- You don't have to rely on laxatives—pills, powders, coffee, or tea.

The Beet Root Test

Eat a bowl full of beets at the start of your cleanse, and note how many days it takes for you to see red (the color of beets) in your stool. Repeat at the end of the cleanse. This can give you an indication of how quickly your food is being digested and passing through your system.

Small children provide a great example of the body as a well-functioning machine. Anyone who's spent any significant amount of time with a 3-year-old has experienced the drill. You sit down for dinner, take one bite of food, and suddenly little Jack exclaims that he needs to go potty! To the skeptical parent, it sounds like a convenient ploy to get out of eating broccoli. But in reality, kids are the perfect example of a healthy elimination system. They go several times a day effortlessly, and as soon as they take one bite of food, the vagus nerve—which conveys sensory information from the body's organs to the central nervous system—sends a signal so strong the child's body immediately knows it's time to go.

Unfortunately, most of us adults no longer experience many of the signs of healthy elimination because we don't have fully functioning digestive systems. But by changing your diet—increasing fiber, adding more greens, reducing or eliminating system-clogging foods—it's possible to very quickly tune things up. Before long, you, too, can have the digestive system of a 3-year-old.

Conscious Success Story: Improving Digestive Function

Past cleanse participant Megan is a 35-year-old mother of four boys. Since high school, she has suffered from significant digestive problems, including regular diarrhea, gas, and bloating. She was seeing a specialist to help with her problems, but with little results or relief. Her next step with her doctor was to start taking medications to help with the pain her digestive issues were causing.

Megan decided that before resorting to a chemical regimen for what she was told could be the rest of her life, she signed up for the cleanse. Amazingly, Megan had never been advised to try changing her diet, and it took mere days for her to reap the benefits.

"The biggest and most important change for me was the huge improvement in my digestion," she explains. "I was just three days in and for the first time since I was a teenager, I wasn't experiencing gas or pain after eating. In fact, I didn't even have cramping—or any of my other usual symptoms—during my period. I'm going to keep wheat, dairy, and tomatoes out of my diet going forward, and I love my green smoothies now! I feel way too good to ever go back."

Battling the Food Demons

Throughout this book, we talk about a lot of things you can do to improve your body's overall efficiencies, but truly nothing plays a more significant role in compromising our collective health than the overconsumption of the "big three" food demons: sugar, gluten, and dairy.

Here's where our biological settings are at odds with the modern world: we are physically drawn to these things—our bodies crave them, and the more we consume, the more we crave—despite the fact that they're cumulatively responsible for a staggering percentage of this country's health challenges. So while we prefer to focus on all the great whole foods available, it's necessary to touch on each of these "food demons" to understand why we keep them off your plate during the Conscious Cleanse and greatly limit their consumption afterward.

The Addictive Power of Sugar

Ah, sugar. We use it to keep us going in our fast-paced lives. We use it to soothe us when we're stressed, sad, or lonely. We use it to celebrate our major life events.

Think about a child at her 1-year-old birthday party. This is often the time when children are given their first taste of sugar. It's really interesting to watch because a small child hasn't developed the taste for the extreme sweetness. She makes a face at the intensity of the sugar, sometimes even pushing it away after the first bite. But food is love, right? We celebrate our sweet moments with sweet tastes, so we, like our parents before us, encourage the child to eat more, to enjoy. And a new food addiction is born.

Sugar, in all its various processed forms, is at the very top of our "food demon" list. It's also, ironically, the one food demon we're not going to completely eliminate during the Conscious Cleanse (but more on that toward the end of this section).

Prevalence of Sugar Sensitivities

According to raw food pioneer David Wolfe, "Many individuals in the Western world are afflicted with hypoglycemia [low blood sugar] and diabetes. Estimates range as high as 40 percent of the population are suffering with hypoglycemia but do not know it. The explosion of adult-onset diabetes also points to chronic mineral deficiencies as well as the overconsumption of hydrogenated oils and refined sugar. Candida is also another form of sugar sensitivity, and nearly everyone with digestive disturbances is suffering from some level of candida." And according to the *American Journal of Preventative Medicine*, 90 percent of people with prediabetes don't even know they have it. Of the ones who do know, only half are actively trying to reduce their risk of full-blown diabetes.

One of the things that makes sugar so dangerous is that it can be found in so many forms and is hidden in so many of our foods. It's everywhere. We often consume it even when we don't know it. It's highly addictive. And much research shows it's nothing short of poison in our systems.

In fact, Dr. Robert Lustig, one of the country's leading experts on childhood obesity, blames an overconsumption of sugar almost exclusively for the explosion of obesity and diabetes—not to mention hypertension, heart disease, and many types of cancer—rampant in our society. Excess sugar, especially refined sugar, has been linked to suppressed immune system, hyperactivity, inability to concentrate, anxiety, depression, ADD/ADHD, premature aging, obesity, arthritis, diabetes, headaches, overeating, mood swings, asthma and allergies, highly acidic blood, inflammation, and insomnia.

It's important to note that sugar's relationship to obesity is not about excess or "empty" calories, according to Lustig. It's much more serious than that. It's about no less than sugar's role in the failure of the body's vital systems. Even synthetic "zero-calorie" sugar substitutes like the ones found in diet sodas can wreak havoc on the body's ability to regulate blood sugar levels. Research has shown that people who consume daily no-calorie sweeteners like aspartame are at increased risk for becoming overweight and developing diabetes.

Manufacturing companies know the highly addictive nature of sugar, and they aren't afraid to use it—hide it, the cynics in us believe—in their products to keep you coming back for more. And it's no side effect of formulating recipes. Food manufacturers do this consciously; it's like built-in marketing. The more you eat, the more you buy, the cheaper they can sell it to you (so you can buy more).

Let's take a look at where the sweet stuff is hiding. We talk a lot about the need to become a "label detective" as you begin preparing your shopping lists, and sugar is one of the best examples of that need. In their book *Suicide by Sugar*, Nancy Appleton and G. N. Jacobs list the various ways sugar can show up on ingredient lists, including the following:

Agave syrup	Honey
Aspartame (artificial)	Invert sugar
Barley malt	Lactose
Beet sugar	Maltose
Cane sugar	Maple syrup
Cane syrup	Molasses
Confectioners' sugar	Raw sugar
Crystalline fructose	Rice syrup
Crystalline sugar	Saccharin (artificial)
Date sugar	Sucanat sugar
Evaporated sugar cane	Sucralose (artificial)
Fructose	Sugarcane syrup
Galactose	Table sugar
Glucose	Turbinado sugar
Granulated sugar	Unrefined sugar
High-fructose corn syrup	White sugar

Even some of the foods people tend to think of as healthy alternatives can have high levels of sugar. This is particularly true of dried fruits. A dried mango, for example, delivers *seven* times the amount of sugar into the bloodstream as a fresh one.

So what is sugar doing in the body that's so harmful? To be clear, the human body needs sugar—more specifically, glucose—to function. So while one of the most important components of the Conscious Cleanse includes a significant reduction of your sugar consumption, you won't fully eliminate all sugars during the program. You'll try to avoid all refined and artificial sugars, certainly, but you'll still get your sweet fix through the natural sugars in fruit (ideally not dried fruit for the reasons already mentioned) and natural sweeteners, in moderation, like stevia, honey, agave, and maple syrup.

Glucose provides your body with energy. It's a power supply to your brain, your muscles, and your organs. You can't survive without it.

The problem is that most of us have a reliance on quick energy in the form of processed and refined sugars, so instead of using our own energy, the body relies on getting it from an outside source. You wake up, and you get an injection of sugar in your processed, sugar-laden cereal. "Yum," your body says as it releases the feel-good neurotransmitter serotonin. The afternoon hits, and with it comes the lows of energy, so you swing by Starbucks for a skinny "sugar free" caramel macchiato. "Yum," your body says again. And the routine continues through bedtime, when you finally fall down from exhaustion. The cycle of peaks and valleys, the highs and lows, the roller coaster of sweet sugar is wreaking havoc on your body.

Physiologically speaking, the problem is an excess of insulin. When you give yourself these hits of sugar, your pancreas has to produce more insulin to control your blood sugar levels. Your body releases the excess insulin into your bloodstream, and this sugar is stored as fat. The result? More fat stored in your cells and your tissues, which translates to a thicker belly, butt, and thighs. It feels impossible to lose weight, because instead of using stored fat for energy, your body is using the quick hit of sugar you give it every couple hours.

Need more reasons to reduce your intake of the stuff? Consuming sugar and excessive sweeteners can feed organisms in your body like bad bacteria, yeast, viruses, Candida, and even mutated cells. Yes, we said *mutated cells*. Here's the deal: when you eat sugar, you run the likely risk of making your body overly acidic. Cancer thrives in an acidic environment! Keep refined sugar off your plate, and keep all sugar intake in check, for the next 2 weeks and see what happens to your energy levels. You may never want—or need—to go back!

Gluten: The Sticky Glue in Your System

The gluten-free rage is sweeping the country. But why? We hear many participants come into the program skeptical that the gluten-free movement is a fad akin to the low-fat or no-carb crazes. Instead of buying into the hype, let's understand what's actually going on.

Gluten is a protein—not a grain—but it is found in wheat, rye, barley, and contaminated oats (oats that are milled in facilities that also mill the aforementioned grains). Because of its gluelike properties, gluten is used as a binder, thickener, and coating.

The primary reason gluten is causing so much trouble is because, like sugar, it is lurking in so much of what we eat. There are the obvious culprits—bread, pizza, pasta, cookies—but this food demon also lurks in foods that may, on the surface, appear to be gluten free, such as barbecue sauce, beer, bread, cereal, condiments, cookies, couscous, crackers, gravies, pasta, salad dressings, semolina, and soy sauce. (For a complete list, go to celiac.com.)

And because of the way wheat is so heavily overmanufactured today, gluten is now released even faster into the bloodstream, causing a roller-coaster effect on your already unstable blood sugar. Further, the very properties that cause it to thicken and bind in the processing of grains also cause it to thicken and bind as it's broken down in your body. It's easy to imagine the same gluelike effect clogging up the works and causing an inflammatory immune response as the body attempts to cope.

In fact, according to a study published in the *New England Journal of Medicine*, gluten has been linked to more than 50 disorders, including autoimmune disease, irritable bowel syndrome, migraines, arthritis, lupus, depression, anxiety, anemia, vitamin D deficiencies, heart disease, cancer, autism, and multiple sclerosis.

Conscious Success Story: The Benefits of Eliminating Gluten

Marissa, 34, has completed the Conscious Cleanse twice and has been maintaining the 80:20 principle (see Part 3) since her first cleanse a year ago. Marissa eliminated gluten and dairy completely and limited sugar and caffeine. After 10 years of visits to doctors, specialists, endocrinologists, acupuncturists, herbalists, and anyone else who would give her an appointment, Marissa's FSH levels were consistently in the premature menopause range. She was told she had ovarian failure and would not be able to get pregnant. After years of hopelessness, weight gain, emotional struggles, and intermittent periods, Marissa was resigned to the fact she could not have babies.

After her second cleanse, Marissa had her yearly FSH test, and her levels were in the normal range. Her tests showed she was, in fact, ovulating normally and no longer in premature menopause. She now has consistent periods, normal weight, and balanced hormonal activity. She's now being told there's no obvious reason why she won't be able to conceive a child if she chooses to do so.

As Marissa excitedly declares, "I know without a doubt that my 'reawakening' is directly related to eliminating gluten through eating the Conscious Cleanse way!"

Contrary to common belief, gluten isn't just something people with celiac disease should avoid. According to leading dietary expert Mark Hyman, MD, "99 percent of people who have a problem with eating gluten don't even know it. They ascribe their ill health or symptoms to something else—not gluten sensitivity—which is 100 percent curable."

Aside from being linked to the onset of multiple diseases, gluten also causes weight gain. As mentioned earlier, it's been shown that gluten can create an inflammatory response in the body. The inflammation results in insulin resistance, so your body has to produce more insulin to regulate the blood sugar in your system. As discussed earlier, insulin is a fat storage hormone, and an overproduction of insulin leads to an overabundance of fat being stored, as opposed to being put to work.

It's important to remember that just because something is gluten free doesn't necessarily mean it's healthy. In fact, many of the processed gluten-free foods contain hidden sugar, fat, and preservatives. A gluten-free cookie is still a cookie!

Not Necessarily Healthy

Gluten free is not synonymous with *healthy*.

When removing gluten from your diet, take the guesswork out of it. Focus on eating whole, unprocessed foods. Think about an apple: one ingredient, and no gluten!

It can be very challenging to be a gluten detective when it comes to packaged foods, so do yourself a favor and steer clear. The best gluten-free products aren't *products* at all!

Do We Really Need Dairy?

Ever stop to consider why humans are the only mammals on the planet who drink milk from a different animal? We are also the only mammals on the planet who continue to consume milk after being weaned from our mothers' breast milk. Think about it. Mammals nurse their young because the milk is dense in nutrients essential to the intense growth curve of babies. As mothers, we fatten up our babies with our milk. Want to pack on the pounds? Drink milk. Load up on cheese and yogurt.

But like the other food demons in this section, the real issue with dairy is actually not about weight gain. Unfortunately, it's more problematic than that.

According to the American Academy of Family Physicians, about 75 percent of adults worldwide are not capable of digesting milk. Beyond childhood, your body stops producing the enzyme needed to break down and digest lactose, the sugar found in milk.

But what about the "Milk: It does a body good" campaign? What about all those health benefits we've been inundated with over the years? Where does the calcium we need come from, if not from milk or cheese?

First of all, studies show that dairy is doing more harm than good in your body. In his book *The China Study*, Dr. T. Colin Campbell points out that research shows countries consuming the most dairy and dairy products have the highest rates of bone fractures and overall bone health. Crazy, isn't it? We're told to drink milk for calcium to strengthen our bones. But when you consume dairy and other animal protein, you actually increase the acidic state of your body. To neutralize the acidic state, your body must pull from its more basic, or alkalizing, reserves—calcium. Your body, in its infinite wisdom, goes to your bones and takes calcium from there. When this happens too often, the result, ironically, is low bone density.

Although we've been taught to believe the best source of calcium comes from milk and cheese, plants are a great source of calcium (and protein, we might add)! Campbell suggests we "eat a variety of plant foods, and avoid animal foods, including dairy. Plenty of calcium is available in a wide range of plant foods, including beans and leafy vegetables."

So back to our original question: What *are* good sources of calcium? The following list offers a few great plant-based sources:

- Almonds
- Brazil nuts
- Broccoli
- Dark leafy greens (collard greens, kale, spinach)
- Flaxseeds
- Kelp
- Nettle leaf tea
- Okra
- Quinoa
- Sesame seeds

Sorry to burst your dairy bubble, but the stats are in. The research is abundantly clear. Consuming milk, cheese, and yogurt as dietary staples does not, in fact, do the body good.

Many of us were raised on dairy, so we now have evidence of the link between the overconsumption of dairy products and allergies. Often, those of us with dairy allergies are more prone to chronic ear infections, diarrhea and bloating, sinus congestion, trouble breathing, asthma, acne, eczema, and frequent colds and infections.

One last fact to consider: dairy is a mucus-forming food. The body produces mucus as a by-product of inflammation, and inflammation, as we have and will continue to mention, is a root cause of disease.

Give up the dairy, and experience what it's like to breathe easier, have clearer skin, and boost your immune system! And don't worry—satisfying alternatives to dairy exist. (We discuss these in the upcoming "Rethinking Your Shopping Cart" chapter.)

What Not to Eat

Eliminating gluten, dairy, and sugar are crucial to improving your health and achieving the desired results during the cleanse, but there's more to the picture. Over the next 2 weeks, you'll also keep certain other foods off your plate, namely alcohol, caffeine, chocolate, corn, dairy (cheese, yogurt, milk, whey protein, butter), eggs, grapefruit, nightshades (potatoes, tomatoes, eggplants, peppers), oranges, peanuts, shellfish, soy (tamari, tofu, tempeh, miso, edamame), squash and sweet potatoes, strawberries, sugar, wheat and gluten products, and yeast and yeasted products.

These foods top the allergen lists. And because we know up to 90 percent of all allergies and sensitivities go undetected, it's an important exercise to explore their effects on you. You may notice a few items on the list, such as squash, sweet potatoes, and potatoes, that aren't generally considered allergens. We included them because they're heavy, starchy vegetables that require more digestive effort, which is exactly what we're hoping to minimize throughout the cleanse.

You might think you don't have an allergy to these foods, but allergens don't just result in your face swelling or your throat closing. Your symptoms could cause your body to become inflamed or your digestive system not to process your food, causing weight gain. But even if you're still convinced you have no allergies, that you never have any negative reaction to food, please humor us. Give it a try as a part of your grand experiment with us. You can do anything for 2 weeks.

Often the foods you crave and love the most are the ones that cause the most damage in your body. Consider a food you can't live without. How often do you consume it? What does it feel like when you think about taking this food off your plate? Consider for a moment that this intense attachment you have to coffee, for example, is the key component to unlocking healing powers within you.

Hiding in Plain Sight

Most food allergies, by their very nature, are masked and hidden. It is hidden from the patient, hidden from his or her family, and hidden from the medical profession in general. It is said that often the solution to a difficult problem is right in front of your nose, but you cannot see it. In the case of food allergies, the source of the problem is literally in front of you, in the form of some commonly eaten substance that is bringing on and per-petuating chronic symptoms .... In my experience, food allergies are one of the greatest health problems in our country.

—Dr. Theron Randolph

We are creatures of habit, and our habits take their toll. Corn, soy, wheat, and sugar fill so much of what's available to us, so we end up consuming the same food at every meal, every day, often without even knowing it. Over time, this overload not only causes an allergy or sensitivity, but it can actually make your body respond to these foods as toxins, ultimately causing the deterioration of your digestive system. Your body can no longer break down these products, and therefore starts to recognize them as toxic. The Conscious Cleanse is designed purposefully to remove as much food toxicity as possible, allowing your body time to rest and repair itself.

We should also note that the earlier list is not exhaustive. There may be other foods you may be sensitive or allergic to, and it's important to be aware of allergens and potential allergens. Jo, for example, cannot tolerate avocados, although they're a healthy food. Any food that causes inflammation or sensitivity in your body can make you sick, cause weight gain, and even cause neurological and emotional disorders! Remember, you are your own best investigator. Be open, listen to your body, and take note of the messages and cues you're sending yourself.

Confused About Soy?

A slew of mixed messages surround this little bean. Many studies support the benefits, suggesting it prevents cancer, lowers cholesterol, and balances hormones. Just as many claim the opposite: soy *causes* breast cancer, blocks thyroid function, causes hyperactivity and panic attacks. Our main concerns with soy lie in the fact that it's genetically modified, which we have yet to discover the real safety of, and it's mucus forming. Soy, like corn, is also lurking in countless processed convenience foods, like salad dressing. Take a break from soy and reintroduce it into your diet after the cleanse, and see how you feel. Forget all the data and inconclusive research, and let your body do the talking.

The Conscious Cleanse Way

Let food be your medicine and medicine be your food.

—Hippocrates of Cos

We often hear from our program participants who feel like they eat what they consider rather healthy diets already. They steer clear of fast food and rarely partake in pizza, fries, chips, or other "junk"; they enjoy an occasional dessert but don't go overboard on sweets; they avoid soda and other sugary beverages. They often feel like they already "know how to eat."

Yet something brings them to the cleanse. The specifics of that "something" vary from person to person, but there's a marked commonality among them, a shared gap. Whether their call is weight loss, digestive issues, illness, general sluggishness, or some undefined need to reboot, each of these people know, at least on a subconscious level, that their bodies are calling for a tune-up.

For some of our participants, the dietary changes we suggest feel more like a tweak than a monumental shift, and yet even those subtle changes can have cumulative effects that are far from subtle. For others, the Conscious Cleanse way of eating is a complete 180 from what they're used to. Either way, there's something inspirational about committing to change, a spark that ignites within us and brings us to life. When we put ourselves in unfamiliar territory, we're forced to come off autopilot and pay attention.

In this chapter, we begin to explore with some more specificity what it means to "eat the Conscious Cleanse way," but at the heart of what we're suggesting is that you begin to play with consciousness. Because ultimately, before you can change what you're doing, you have to notice what you're doing in the first place.

Conscious Success: Waking Up to Life

Kate is a busy mother of two. When we first met her as a participant at one of our seminars, she was juggling a demanding full-time job with her responsibilities at home and fitting in time for herself as a last, and often overlooked, priority. She described herself as "pretty normal and pretty happy." She told us she made time to exercise two or three times a week, often having to wake up at unseemly hours to do so. She tried to eat a relatively healthy diet, very rarely partaking in anything she considered an overindulgence. She'd wanted to try a cleanse for a while, she told us, but kept finding reasons to put it off, mostly due to her schedule and responsibilities.

Focus on What You Want

Where the attention goes, energy flows. Put your thoughts on what you want, and when thoughts that don't serve that purpose come up, notice them and go back to what you *do* want (to be pain free, for example) or what you *do* get to eat.

The rush of getting herself ready for work and her kids ready for school in the morning often meant she didn't have time for breakfast other than a cup of coffee. She'd have another cup at work, and often got so busy she wouldn't realize she hadn't eaten until 1 or 2 o'clock, at which time she'd grab "something quick," always fighting the urge for a heavy carbohydrate fix—and winning the fight more often than not. Another cup of coffee or a few bites from the candy bowl in the office helped get her through the afternoon slump.

Dinner for the family consisted of something "fast and easy," although she'd try to keep it as healthy as possible: a grab-and-go chicken from the supermarket's hot case, takeout Chinese food (steering clear of the fried stuff), or some boiled pasta and jarred spaghetti sauce. There was always a vegetable on the side. Sometimes a modest dessert: a celebratory cookie, a small cup of ice cream. A glass of wine after the kids went to bed.

Kate didn't suffer any major health issues. She got migraine headaches from time to time, which she attributed to stress at work. She fought off colds all winter, which she attributed to having two kids in school. She had hay fever in the spring, which she attributed to the luck of the draw. She had a sore neck and back, which she attributed to natural aging and sitting at the computer all day. She didn't consider herself "fat" by any stretch, but she had an extra 10 pounds she couldn't seem to shake after her second child's birth.

Her final motivation to join the Conscious Cleanse was that she had planned a beach vacation, and she was hoping she could lose a few pounds to feel more comfortable in her bathing suit. As Kate describes it, "I came in to get ready for my vacation, and ended up finding a true journey within my everyday life."

Kate lost her 10 pounds ("12, to be exact") during her cleanse, but more than that, she describes:

"I stopped missing my coffee after the first week—and I *loved* my coffee. I wasn't tired at the end of the workday. Or at least the 'tired' I felt, felt different. I started sleeping more deeply than I had in years and waking up more refreshed.

"Meals became a little adventure—our family explored together, we experimented. Even when the experiment failed, it was an experience you just don't get over take-out Chinese. We still laugh about 'the beet quinoa debacle.' Throughout the cleanse, I never felt hungry, never felt like I was depriving myself. I felt like I was 'doing something' as opposed to the other diets I've tried, where it was about '*not* doing something.' Somewhere in the middle of the program I came to a kind of profound realization. I'd just tweaked my habits and my perspective, let go of what I was used to—just a little. There was almost no willpower involved. But in those seemingly small changes, something significant happened for me.

"Toward the end of the cleanse, I realized I hadn't had a headache in a while, that my constantly stuffy nose was totally unobstructed. My neck stopped aching. I rediscovered my libido, which got my husband's attention. (He actually ended up doing the next cleanse with me!) Not to mention the weight loss, which just seemed effortless. It seems corny to admit, but I felt suddenly … awake."

We hear some version of this story with astounding frequency. Even if we think we're eating a comparatively healthful diet, we suffer myriad "common, everyday ailments." We tell ourselves our aches and pains and minor ailments are all a part of getting older or "just in my DNA." Can it be possible that we're telling ourselves lies?

The New Normal

A big part of the problem is that we're getting mixed messages. The white noise is relentless: the 24-hour news cycle, the mass marketing machines of big food companies, the constant churn of fad diets, commercials, infomercials, product placement, studies that contradict studies that contradict studies. Does a cup of coffee every morning prevent cancer or cause Parkinson's this week? Am I supposed to eliminate fat or count calories or weigh my food or subsist on bacon alone? Can I really reduce my risk of diabetes by changing cereal brands? Whole grain, gluten free, fat free, low fat, trans fats, all natural, low sodium, low carb, low sugar, enhanced, enriched …

It's as clichéd as it is true to say: you are what you eat. The problem is that these days, it can be next to impossible to know what we're actually eating. So what are we? In so many important ways, we've lost our connection to the very thing that sustains us. And it's because, quite simply and quite understandably, we don't know what to believe any more. And who can blame us?

You Are What You Eat

Quite literally, you are what you eat. Think about it: your body processes the food you eat and it literally becomes your tissues, cells, bones, and muscles. Consider that the next time you're craving a hot dog.

Do any of these sound familiar: headaches or migraines, chronic pain (mild or otherwise), weight gain or obesity, constipation, gas, seasonal allergies, regular colds, thyroid issues, insomnia, fatigue, exhaustion, depression, stress, clogged sinuses, acne, high cholesterol, high blood pressure, dandruff, itchy scalp, dry skin, gout, Crohn's disease, or irregular menstruation or infertility? The list, of course, goes on.

Is this the new reality? Is it "normal" to have chronic aches and pains, to sneeze and cough through every cold or allergy season, to "need" three cups of coffee to keep going through the day? Is it "normal" to feel regularly tired and generally unfulfilled? If "normal" means "common," then yes, all those things are normal. But the fact is, that version of normal is *not necessary*. It's possible—and best of all, it's ultimately *easy*—to set the bar higher, to expect more, to create a new normal for yourself.

The guiding principles of the Conscious Cleanse may seem hidden amidst the chaos of all the competing messages these days, but ultimately, what we hear most often from cleanse participants is how simple these principles are, how obvious they seem once they're applied—and how quickly and drastically they improve general well-being.

As you'll see in the sections that follow, the Conscious Cleanse is about a return to simplicity. It's about creating a fresh start, decluttering, and getting back to basics—cleaning up by stripping down. It is, at heart, about reconnecting with the thriving, healing, fundamental you.

Celebrating Whole Foods

The North Star of the Conscious Cleanse lies in a very simple principle:

> Eat whole foods.

So what's a whole food? Start by imagining a food's origins. Does it come from a living thing? Can you picture it growing in a field or on a tree or in the ocean? Whole foods are foods that do not *have* ingredients—they *are* the ingredient. They're often the items that exist on the periphery of the grocery store and they are the colorful foods that fill farmers' markets. A piece of broccoli, for example, is a whole food. A Cheez-It snack cracker is not. Simple, right?

Whole foods often don't have packaging or labels. Whole foods have a shelf life and will spoil if they're not eaten within a short period of time. Whole foods generally aren't advertised on television. Whole foods are foods like fresh fruits, herbs, vegetables, nuts, seeds, grains, and legumes, and also can include natural unprocessed cuts of meat, fish, and poultry.

As the new normal of the "Conscious Cleanse way" becomes second nature, should you find yourself standing in the grocery store pondering whether a certain food is indeed a whole food, ask yourself how that food exists in nature. Generally, if you can imagine the food's origins, you can easily determine whether it's a whole food.

A good example is rice. We have had a number of cleanse participants ask about brown rice pasta. While this certainly is a healthy alternative to the traditional white flour pasta, it's still not considered a whole food. Think for a moment of rice growing in a paddy. You can picture what a grain of rice looks like, right? But can you imagine a plant with long, slippery noodles growing from it? Nope. Not even in Italy.

Whole Food or Not?

Brown rice, chicken deli meat, apples, veggie straws, fresh fruit salad, quinoa pasta, rice cakes, raw vegetables, fruit leather, chicken breasts, applesauce, quinoa—how many of these do you think are whole foods? You might be surprised at the answers: brown rice—yes; chicken deli meat—no; apples—yes; veggie straws—no; fresh fruit salad—yes; quinoa pasta—no; rice cake—no; raw vegetables—yes; fruit leather—no; chicken breasts—yes; applesauce—no; quinoa—yes.

Exploring Raw and Living Foods

While the basis of the Conscious Cleanse is whole foods, it's important to go a step further when talking about fresh fruits and vegetables. You may be familiar with the "raw food movement," in which eating 100 percent raw food, or food that hasn't been heated past 118°F, is revered for its disease-curing and life-affirming properties.

At its core, the Conscious Cleanse seeks to bridge the gap between this somewhat challenging way of eating and a realistically accessible and sustainable standard—a middle ground, if you will.

Raw and living foods include uncooked fruits, vegetables, nuts, seeds, and sprouted grains and beans (for more information on sprouts, see Day 6). These foods are not processed, heated, cooked, or altered in any way. They are the pure essence of whole food in its natural state.

Going Raw

Raw, living food provides high-quality nourishment. We are all aware of the vitamin and mineral value of uncooked fruits and vegetables, but most of us are unaware that raw food has much more to offer—vital food enzymes. The food enzymes in raw food predigest food in our stomachs [and are] the key to a long, healthy life without disease.

—*The Hippocrates Diet and Health Program* by Ann Wigmore

So what's the big deal about raw and living foods? In one word, *enzymes*. Enzymes are your body's sparkplugs. Every action your body performs, from blinking your eyes to digesting your food, requires an enzymatic reaction. When you ingest foods that don't contain enzymes, your body uses its own enzymes to properly break down the food into absorbable nutrients. Raw and living foods are chock-full of these enzymes. The catch is that these enzymes are, as you may have guessed, heat sensitive. The more the food is cooked, the fewer of its enzymes survive, and the more your body has to use its own enzymes to break down the food.

Two additional concepts point to the benefits of increasing raw foods in your diet. The first of these concepts originated from a study on the effects of food and our immune systems conducted under the direction of Dr. Paul Kouchakoff (Institute of Clinical Chemistry in Lausanne, Switzerland, 1930). The alarming results of the study showed that when we eat cooked foods, our bodies respond by raising white blood cell counts, as if the body is actually defending against a foreign body or infection.

The study also found that the most dramatic response was produced by refined processed foods like white flour and white rice, pasteurized products like milk, and preserved foods containing chemicals that increase shelf life. Conversely, eating uncooked, raw, unaltered whole foods did not produce the same bodily response.

The second concept deals with the amount of time and energy it takes the body to properly break down, digest, and absorb nutrients from food. In addition to requiring enzymes, our bodies need energy to digest and absorb food. When we eat a diet rich in raw, living food, our bodies use half to one third of the energy required to digest a cooked, standard American meal. Imagine what you might do with this extra energy.

Think about how you feel after a huge, indulgent meal. Are you more "get up and go" or "lay down and groan"? Like every outward symptom you feel, this "food coma syndrome" begins at a cellular level. When your body isn't entirely focused on digesting that last meal, it has excess energy to devote to a deeper maintenance and healing of the liver, kidneys, pancreas, and gallbladder, as well as other bodily functions.

What's amazing about this is that without even realizing it, we're able to cleanse our cells, release fat from tissues, and tune up our other organs so they can work more efficiently. And the results are nothing short of astonishing.

Chronic pain disappears, stubborn pounds melt away, fine lines fade, skin looks brighter, eyesight improves, memory improves, and sleep is more restful. At the deepest levels, our mental clarity becomes sharper, we tune into intuition, and we make once-challenging decisions more easily and with absolute certainty. Confidence and a sense of well-being are literally built from the inside out.

During the Conscious Cleanse, we encourage participants to eat raw or lightly steamed vegetables. If you've been eating a mostly cooked diet, you can easily transition to lightly steamed veggies that are both warming and easy to digest. For people who haven't eaten a lot of raw food, it can actually be difficult on the system initially. Stick with it, and your system will adjust. Don't be afraid of baby steps, of experimentation. Focus first on lightly steaming your vegetables, and try integrating more raw and living foods over a period of time. That way you'll still get many of the live enzymes *and* your body will be able to more easily digest it. It's like having your cake and eating it, too—only without the cake.

Why Enzymes Rule

When food is heated to 118°F or higher, food enzymes are destroyed. The result is that the body has to work harder to produce its own enzymes to break down and assimilate the cooked or processed food. Food that's been pasteurized (as in most bottled juices), canned, or microwaved is deficient in natural enzymes. A diet rich in raw food is not only rich in enzymes, it's also rich in minerals, which helps the body turn to its own enzyme stores, resulting in more energy and a supercharged immune system.

Throughout the cleanse, it's important to start where you are, to practice forgiving yourself for any perceived "missteps." No part of the journey you're about to embark on is all or nothing. Even Gabriel Cousens, founder of the Tree of Life Rejuvenation Center and long-time expert on raw and living food and holistic healing, explains that we get the same benefits from eating an 80 percent plant-based living food diet as we would from eating a 100 percent living food diet.

We believe this is a more flexible, compassionate, and less-rigid approach than trying to maintain a 100 percent raw food diet. And if you're going from 0 percent to 20 percent or from 20 percent to 40 percent, you will be making vast improvements that you'll recognize quickly and be able to sustain.

So let's set aside the labels and the percentages all together and keep it simple. Infuse your body with as much raw and living food as possible, and you'll be well on your way. Focus on eating nutrient-dense foods instead of counting calories and fat grams. Learn to eat intuitively, listening to your body rather than whatever fad diet is being featured on the morning news.

Beware Packaging and Labels

We've already defined whole foods as foods that exist in nature and have not been altered from their original state. But you'll quickly find that it's not all as easy as choosing between broccoli and Cheez-Its. As with anything, shades of gray flank the black and white, so it's worth exploring ways to make good, "clean" choices when things start to get murky during the cleansing and detoxifying process.

Many whole foods can be purchased in the bulk section of your local grocery or health food store—things like nongluten grains, legumes, and raw (unroasted and unsalted) nuts and seeds. The other mainstay of the cleanse diet is, as we've mentioned, raw vegetables and fruits; again, no special or fancy packaging is necessary.

What about sauces, dressings, and dips? Fear not: you'll be far from a flavorless existence during the Conscious Cleanse. And while we encourage participants to make these items from scratch whenever possible, we do provide some suggestions for brands we know and trust in the shopping list in the "Rethinking Your Shopping Cart" chapter.

The goal, ultimately, is to keep your food intake as "clean" as possible during the Conscious Cleanse. Stay *conscious* about what you're eating—a difficult task amid aisles and aisles of marketing messages. Difficult, maybe. Time consuming, certainly. But not impossible. Invest a little bit of time, and you'll be amazed at what you learn in 2 short weeks.

Jules shares a story about her discovery of sunflower seed butter to show the importance of label examination. With the onset of her second pregnancy, she found her body suddenly requiring more protein than it had before, and nut butters became a staple of her pregnancy diet. At first glance, a particular brand of sunflower seed butter looked like a clean alternative to her regular raw almond butter, but for some reason, she caught herself overindulging in it, craving it constantly—to the point where she saw it as a kind of addiction.

Jules knew true whole foods don't cause this kind of compulsion, so she did a little label investigation and saw that, indeed, the second ingredient next to roasted sunflower seeds was "organic cane juice." Organic cane juice? What the heck is that? And how is it that you can read a label and still not understand exactly what's in the product you're ingesting? Jules switched back to her raw almond butter and quickly found that, once again, she didn't overindulge. She would eat just enough to feel satisfied, and that was that. No going back to the fridge for second or third spoonfuls. Turns out, organic cane juice is actually just sugar, slightly less processed than good old-fashioned white sugar, but sugar nonetheless.

The point is—we've said it before, and we'll say it again—become a label detective! Whole books have been written on this topic alone. (Our favorite is *Eating Between the Lines* by Kimberly Lord Stewart, most easily found as an ebook.) Keep it simple, slow it down, and start to pay attention to what you're actually eating.

In a nutshell, when purchasing anything packaged, read the label carefully. The fewer ingredients, the better. And if you see something on the list you (or a third grader) can't pronounce, keep it out of your grocery basket. (Unless it's quinoa—why is that word pronounced *KEEN-wah?*—but you get the point!)

The cleaner you keep your food, the fewer complications you're likely to encounter. Just because a product says it's "gluten free" or "USDA organic" or "kosher" or "vegan" doesn't mean it's a perfect whole food, nor does it ensure you're getting a "clean" product.

Exceptions to the clean food list (that do come in a package) are things like olive oil, flaxseed oil, apple cider vinegar, Ume plum vinegar, honey, tahini, raw almond butter, sea vegetables, vegetable or chicken broth, and unsweetened almond milk. See the shopping list section at the end of the "Rethinking Your Shopping Cart" chapter for more details on suggested clean products.

Be a Label Detective

Pick up a few packaged items that look relatively healthy—a can of diced tomatoes, red kidney beans, and applesauce, for example. Now read the ingredient lists. Diced peeled tomatoes: cut tomatoes, tomato juice, calcium chloride, citric acid. Red kidney beans: soaked red kidney beans, water, salt, calcium chloride, disodium EDTA. Organic cinnamon applesauce: organic apples, organic apple juice concentrate, water, ascorbic acid, organic cinnamon. What *are* these things? Calcium chloride is a preservative also used to clear ice from roadways. Citric acid is a natural preservative that's been reported to cause bleaching and skin irritation. Disodium EDTA is a preservative that can become carcinogenic when reacting with other common compounds. Apple juice concentrate is another way to say sugar.

Water, Water Everywhere!

Most people don't drink enough water. Change this one practice, and watch everything else start to fall into place. We keep talking about going back to basics (and we're not going to stop!), and water is as basic as it gets.

Fereydoon Batmanghelidj, MD, a leading professional in water research, says, "Health care in America is in crisis because the professionals and public don't know when the human body is thirsty. Once we understand the thirst mechanism of the body, once we understand the cries of the body for water, 60 percent of the health-care crisis will disappear." That's a huge claim, but the fact of the matter is that most of us actually live a life of chronic dehydration. Some signs that you're not drinking enough water include dry skin, cracked lips, and yellow urine. You also don't produce enough body fluids, you're constipated, and you're tired.

Chronic Dehydration

By the time we feel thirsty, we're already dehydrated. And studies show that a lifetime of regular dehydration accumulates, catching up in the form of allergies and disease.

Water helps with our histamine response and is a natural anti-inflammatory. And according to Mark Hyman, MD, "almost every modern disease is caused or affected by hidden inflammation." In fact, studies have linked increased water intake to improvements in, among other things, chronic pain, asthma, allergic reactions, arthritis, neck and back pain, headaches, stress, depression, cholesterol levels, blood pressure, diabetes, and obesity.

Studies aside, if you practice drinking water during the Conscious Cleanse—and probably significantly more than you're currently drinking—you'll witness the change yourself.

So how much water should you drink? There's no exact formula, so err on the side of more is more! The easiest formula for determining how much water you should focus on consuming in a day is this:

½ your body weight in ounces

For example, if you weigh 150 pounds, your goal should be to drink approximately 75 ounces of water per day. Add an additional 25 ounces if you live at altitude or exercise rigorously. It's also important to drink pure filtered water whenever possible.

We love beginning the day with 36 ounces of warm water with lemon. If you're currently a coffee drinker, we know you won't believe this now, but you might actually be surprised at how readily this warm water concoction can become your go-to morning beverage. Go ahead, keep laughing—it's amazing what a couple weeks of open-mindedness can do.

Lastly, and crucially, your body often confuses thirst for hunger because they can both trigger the same reaction in the brain. Not consuming enough water can actually cause you to consume too much food instead and thus gain weight!

Experiment with a Diet Free of Allergens

An important aspect to the Conscious Cleanse we touch on throughout this book is the allergen-free menu plan. To fully detoxify and reset your system, it's important to embrace this concept of eating an "allergen-free diet" during your Conscious Cleanse journey.

You may wonder, as you build your cleanse menu, why we ask you to avoid things like milk products, eggs, tomatoes, or oranges. The reason for this becomes most obvious during the reintegration phase of the cleanse. Not only is it good to give your system a rest from the foods you tend to enjoy on a regular basis, it's also a key component to you understanding how these foods might be quietly affecting you, and ultimately, to help you determine your ideal diet going forward.

Why No Nightshades?

Nightshades—tomatoes, potatoes, bell peppers, and eggplant—are a diverse class of foods. The problem with eating nightshades during the cleanse is that they contain alkaloids, which can be responsible for joint inflammation in some people. They've been shown to potentially block enzyme activity in those who are alkaloid sensitive. Like all the foods we suggest you keep off your plate, taking a break from a favorite food, like roma tomatoes, for example, can let your body heal in ways you may never have dreamed possible.

At the end of the Conscious Cleanse, you'll have a very unique opportunity to do a mini-experiment with yourself, to isolate your favorite foods in your system, taking note of how each one feels in your body. You may discover that a seemingly harmless component of your regular diet is what's causing your insomnia. Or you may discover you get gas when you eat soy sauce. Can you live with that from time to time? Is an occasional cup of ice cream worth the effect it might have on your system? That's up to you. The point is you'll be empowered by your dietary choices, once and for all.

Conscious Success Story: Learning Something New

Daniel, a self-proclaimed foodie, already followed what he considered a healthy diet, and the Conscious Cleanse was his first experience with a guided nutritional program. Daniel had no symptoms of food allergies going into the program. He viewed the cleanse as a kind of break from all the holiday excess he'd indulged in and describes his experience with the program as "straightforward and not too hard to follow."

His biggest revelation came not during the 2 weeks of the cleanse, but after it was over, during the reintegration phase. Daniel ate a corn tortilla, and shortly after, his neck and face broke out in a rash. Previously, Daniel had not even considered the possibility that he had a sensitivity to corn.

Now, armed with this information, Daniel considers himself more capable of making healthy food choices. He hasn't decided to give up corn products altogether, but he knows there's a mild hindrance when he chooses to partake, and he's better able to weigh his food choices.

Eat When You're Hungry

When did this simple practice become so difficult? We're literally born knowing to eat when we're hungry and stop eating when we're not. It should be one of the simplest, most innate aspects of our existence, shouldn't it?

But for so many of us, that's not how it's done. We've been trained—and in turn train our children—to eat by the clock, even if we had a huge meal just a few hours prior. We've even learned to "get hungry" based on the time of day. We eat empty calories, mindlessly. Mull that one over for a second: we consume that which we don't need, and often don't even *want*, without even thinking about it.

We eat out of convenience. We eat to be polite. We eat because we might not get a chance to eat later. We eat when we're stressed out. We eat when we're bored. We eat after we've had a long day of work. We eat to comfort ourselves, reward ourselves, punish ourselves, or busy ourselves. How often do we actually eat to *nourish* ourselves?

During the Conscious Cleanse, you'll spend 2 weeks focusing on mindfulness, but there's one huge thing you can happily forget about: counting. You'll be liberated from the obsession over calories, fat grams, or protein grams. You'll be feeding your body what it needs, and you'll quickly find that it doesn't want more than that. It's amazing what your body tells you when you stop and listen.

The Conscious Cleanse is the first step to reclaiming the true purpose of your food, to regaining the innate ability to eat for nourishment. Mindful mindlessness. Chew on that.

This is perhaps the most interesting part of the experiment you're about to embark upon. So many of our participants come in skeptical, fearful about eating too much and gaining weight. As modern humans, we've spent a lot of years training ourselves to think this way—it's no wonder we cling to it. For 2 weeks, we invite you to let it go. Forget about what you're used to, reason with your compulsions, and listen to your body on a deeper level.

A New Way of Thinking

Instead of thinking about food in terms of calories or fat grams, start thinking about it in terms of nutrients. Before you eat something, ask yourself, *How nutrient-dense is this food?*

Eating when you're hungry first implies that you have to allow yourself to feel hunger again. Don't be afraid of that statement. It doesn't mean you're going to suffer, and it doesn't mean you're going to starve. *Hunger*, for our purposes, should not have a negative connotation at all. Hunger is not about depriving yourself or restricting yourself. Rather, it's about listening to yourself, learning to give yourself what you need. This tweak in thinking is nothing short of transformative. Slowly, you begin to realize that you actually *want* what it is you *need*. Eventually, you can even feel good about your indulgences. Guilt and remorse go out the door. These are not emotions that belong with food.

Along those same lines, you'll focus on training yourself to eat slowly and mindfully during the Conscious Cleanse—a crucial component of vibrant health. Think of all the European countries where people consume more butter, more croissants, more cheese, and more pasta than we do, and where those same people as a whole suffer far less obesity and heart disease.

The core difference between our cultures is how we traditionally eat. In those European cultures, a 4-hour meal is not uncommon. Dining is an event you share with loved ones, rich with decadent foods and heartfelt conversation. Food is actually *tasted* during these types of meals, and the body is given a chance to respond. There is indulgence, but not *overindulgence.*

While at our dinner tables, it often feels like a race to the finish line. As parents, we shovel food in our faces, ever anticipating our kids' next needs. We tell ourselves we don't have time to sit and enjoy a long meal with the family, and neither they nor we would even know how to approach that type of meal.

Later in the program we delve deeper into these concepts and help guide you through a specific process to explore why you eat, how you eat, and when you eat.

Eat What You Like, and Eat It Joyfully

The Conscious Cleanse is not about restriction, deprivation, calorie control, or dogma. The program is designed for you to start within your comfort zone; make small, often subtle changes along the way; and reap what are often shockingly substantial benefits. It's also designed as a process, allowing you to explore new boundaries within that comfort zone. Each trip through the Conscious Cleanse reveals new health benefits, new foods, and new flavors.

About the Wagon

Remember, in the Conscious Cleanse there is no wagon, so there's no wagon to fall off.

Be flexible! Rigidity is boring and unsustainable. Play with the recipes. Swap out this for that, play with spices and herbs, and experiment with cooking techniques.

Food is joy, and eating should always be joyful—and not just in the fleeting moments while the food is in your mouth. It can be easy to confuse feeding compulsion with feeding hunger. But something that "tastes good going down" and then leaves you feeling bloated or sluggish or sick or guilty or regretful is not joyful.

When we shift our attention away from the foods, and habits, that make us sick, we find an abundance of variety—fresh, wholesome foods that create true vibrancy. Eating what you like is about finding more and more foods that taste good to you; satisfy you; *and* make you feel good, energized, and alive. Be curious and adventurous. Try foods you've never tried before. You may be surprised to find that something you never gave a second glance to at the grocery store can become a new favorite.

A funny thing happens when you clean out your system: your tastes actually begin to change. Your cravings shift. You become attracted to nourishment rather than drawn to physical addictions. What you want is no longer in direct opposition to what you need. And finally, you can believe your appetite again.

Preparing to Cleanse

Before everything else, getting ready is the secret of success.

—Henry Ford

If you take the time to prepare, the Conscious Cleanse is very easy. Physical preparation—things like having your shopping done and prepping meals and snacks beforehand—lead to emotional preparation, so you're not left fighting urges for a quick fix.

In this chapter, we look at the most efficient ways to prepare for the Conscious Cleanse so neither time constraints nor a loss of convenience get in the way of your success. Good preparation helps you remove the guesswork as you step out of your comfort zone, making it all the more comfortable to be there.

Choosing a Time to Begin

Many participants in our programs have concern about timing their cleanse so it doesn't interfere with the things that sometimes get in the way of traditional diets: birthdays, anniversaries, weddings, work travel, exams, and various other scheduled events. *Maybe it's not the right time*, they think. *I don't want to set myself up for failure.*

Here's what we've learned for sure: if you wait for the perfect time, you'll never find it, because it doesn't exist. The time is *now*.

Put away all the reasons this isn't an ideal time. Pull out your calendar. Mark off 2 weeks. Yes, you should probably avoid doing the formal program on your tropical beach vacation or during your twentieth wedding anniversary, but we will show you how to do this program while continuing to live your life. With some preparation, you can go out to restaurants, you can be social, you can travel, and you can still eat the "Conscious Cleanse way."

Of course, the advantage of doing the cleanse on your own time with this book as opposed to our online, phone, or in-person guided programs is that you have flexibility in your timing. But don't put it off! Move it to the top of your to-do list. You're reading this chapter, so that's a great start. Let's begin planning now. What does your next month look like? Ride the wave of your excitement, and commit to a date.

Here are some suggestions for choosing your start date:

Think about the time you're reading this book and prepping for the Conscious Cleanse as part of your program. Think about integrating small aspects of the book as you learn them. Practice is part of preparation, and the more you practice these principles, the smoother a transition into the cleanse you'll have. (Hopefully you're not eating a slice of pizza while you're reading!)

Consider starting the cleanse on a Monday. Days 6 and 7 and days 13 and 14 are "purification days." On these days, we guide you through trying some deeper liquid-, veggie-, and fruit-only cleansing principles. Consider these "rest days." It will absolutely help if you can relax as much as possible during this time, and weekends can be an ideal time for this. Additionally, it may be easier to do your shopping for the week over the weekend before the cleanse. But by no means should you let these suggestions delay you!

Try to avoid the very obvious challenges, but don't sweat the everyday stuff. Thanksgiving might not be the best time to start; dinner with the Johnsons or the business trip to Chattanooga can be managed.

Write it down. Mark the whole 2 weeks on your calendar, and start looking forward to a transformative experience.

Recruit a Partner

We've found that it's very helpful to enroll a friend or family member to do the cleanse with you. Creating a buddy system or a system of support helps you stay on track and committed to a healthier you. If you live with someone—a spouse or a roommate, for example—it makes shopping and preparing meals that much easier. Plus, it's rewarding to share and compare your experiences and results with each other!

It's important to know that regardless of your circumstances, you won't have to suffer through your daily routine on the cleanse. In fact, you'll likely start feeling the benefits right away. So if you're traveling for work, you'll feel sharper and more clearheaded. If you're studying for an exam, you'll have more energy, mental clarity, and the ability to remember things. If you're at a wedding or special event, you'll be deeply present in the company of the people you're with and will have something interesting to talk about. (Not to mention, you'll look great!)

So pull out your calendar right now and write "Day #1 of the Conscious Cleanse." Seriously, go do it before you read any further.

Welcome to the beginning of the rest of your life!

Mapping Your Personal Cleanse

Think about the information we present in the coming pages as a road map. There's more than one route to your destination, and the map allows for detours and variable speeds. The map suggests the scenic route—the one that offers the best views and the most interesting scenery.

Instead of some rigid do-exactly-this-or-you-will-fail diet plan, the Conscious Cleanse offers the framework for you to be your own best healer and teacher. The cleanse is specifically designed to be accessible to just about everyone, under any circumstance, on any budget. This may sound like a lofty ideal, but we've seen it work time and time again with countless and diverse participants.

The key distinction of the Conscious Cleanse can be summed up in one (hyphenated) word: *bio-individuality*. Bio-individuality is a concept first asserted by Dr. Roger J. Williams in his book *Biochemical Individuality*, stating that every single part of the human body, down to the cellular level, is unique, personal, and *individualized* to that person. If no two of us are exactly alike, why would our ideal meal plans be? The Conscious Cleanse recognizes that everyone naturally and bio-chemically has individualized nutritional needs.

In this context, it makes a lot of sense why so many people who follow the latest and greatest fad diet to the letter invariably lose weight only to gain back even more. Not only is this "yo-yo effect" unhealthy, it's also emotionally self-defeating. It creates self-perpetuating feelings of personal failure and sets us up for the downward spiral. It's never the diet's fault. It's always ours. We didn't try hard enough. Our willpower wasn't strong enough. The Conscious Cleanse turns that old and out-of-date concept upside down.

Here's the thing: our bio-individuality is based on our differing ancestries, blueprints, doshas, preferences, blood types, metabolisms, habits, comfort zones, and even, perhaps, our mind-sets. So doesn't it make good sense, if we're starting at different places and our desired destinations are just as diverse, that we have to consider there's no one-size-fits-all solution? Doesn't it make more sense that we select, based on our individual blueprint, an appropriate track to run on, and that we give ourselves the flexibility to change that track as we continue to learn more about ourselves?

Our bodies are sophisticated bio-computers programmed to know what they need to sustain themselves. But first we have to clean the hard drive and remove the viruses. In more concrete terms, that means quieting the mind, clearing out old toxins, and beginning to pay attention to what we're *really* craving for nourishment.

Where Are You Now?

The Conscious Cleanse is designed as a 14-day cleanse program, but you may have gathered by now that it's also, at its core, about making long-lasting changes. The way to sustainable and vibrant health is to take things slowly, one step at a time.

With that in mind, we've created a baseline program that's adjustable to suit your individual needs. We offer alternatives at almost every step. There's no such thing as "doing it right"; there's only "doing it right *for you*."

Along the way, you'll benefit from side trips and experimentations. Just like no two people are the same, no two days are the same. Your needs are likely to change with the seasons, with your levels of physical exertion, and with your hormones. A starting point is just a starting point, so don't overthink it. Remember, this isn't a competition (with yourself or anyone else). We promise you'll begin to see fabulous results by starting where you are. This is key to long-lasting, sustainable results.

The following quick test will help you get thinking about where to start as you move into the Conscious Cleanse. Which of these statements best describes your current health condition or food preferences?

1. I love a good steak, eat chicken as a healthy alternative, and know I should eat more vegetables. I don't function without my protein.

2. I love carbs but try to eat more healthful alternatives like yogurt and cheese. I love a good egg-and-cheese bagel sandwich and try to have at least some fresh fruits and vegetables (salad) every day.

3. I love a fruit-filled smoothie with protein powder. I eat salads every day and am bored with the same old "healthy" options out there. I'm stuck in a rut, and because of convenience, I eat the same foods most people around me eat.

In all likelihood, none of these statements perfectly describes you, but pick one based on your gut feeling, and go from there.

If you identify most with statement #1, maybe you carry a few extra pounds and have tried your share of diets—or even cleanses—in the past. You came out of the gates on those diets strong and determined … and have fallen off them with equal resolve. You may have experienced a variety of health challenges, even if they're mild or you consider them "tolerable"—things like high cholesterol, heartburn, or acid reflux.

If this is you, try supplementing from the base plan with the protein options, when offered. Remember, though, this isn't the Atkins Diet. Don't give yourself a free pass to eat bacon for breakfast, lunch, and dinner. We may all be different, but we can say with confidence that's not good for anyone. If your body craves protein, feed it what it needs. Keep your comfort zone in mind, and continue to push the boundaries of that zone.

Here's a sample meal plan for the "meat lover":

> **Begin the day:** Drink 1 quart warm lemon water.
>
> **Breakfast:** Try 1 quart Coco for Cilantro Smoothie.
>
> **Lunch:** Enjoy a Golden Beet Salad with Basic Broiled Organic Chicken Breast.
>
> **Dinner:** Eat a medley of steamed veggies, including zucchini, broccoli, carrots, and kale, served with Ginger Broiled Salmon.
>
> **Snack:** Carrots and celery sticks dipped in almond butter *or* leftover chicken breast from lunch should do the trick.
>
> **End the day:** Sip at least 8 ounces warm lemon water.

If statement #2 best describes your inclinations, you're probably moderately health-conscious, but you know some of your food choices and habits aren't serving you. At the same time, you don't feel the need to make any extreme dietary changes; you just need help getting back on track. You may have some minor health challenges or have a few pounds to lose, but your energy levels can swing drastically throughout the day.

You'll want to take a look at the grain options when presented. Surprisingly, a "sweet tooth" is often the body's way of signaling it needs more energy. Whole grains are a great way to give the body usable, sustainable energy without spiking the blood sugar and curbing sugar cravings.

Here's a sample meal plan for grain lovers:

> **Begin the day:** Drink 1 quart warm lemon water.
>
> **Breakfast:** Eat some Simple Breakfast Porridge.
>
> **Lunch:** Enjoy a Super Big Easy Salad.
>
> **Dinner:** Try Curried Carrot Soup over 1 cup quinoa with a small green salad and East Meets West Salad Dressing.
>
> **Snack:** Nosh on ½ cup raw walnuts, raw pumpkin seeds, and raw sunflower seeds.
>
> **End the day:** Sip at least 8 ounces warm lemon water.

If statement #3 best describes you, the idea of doing a cleanse might seem like no big deal, and you're ready to jump in with both feet. You're ready to embrace a diet of 75 to 80 percent raw foods but look forward to the occasional piece of fish or a cup of brown rice with your veggies when it's cold outside. You're familiar with myriad detox symptoms and have successfully given up coffee and/or sweets from time to time in the past. You're ready for a challenge and looking for big results.

If that sounds like you, here's your sample meal plan:

> **Begin the day:** Drink 1 quart warm lemon water.
>
> **Breakfast:** Sip 1 quart Green Goddess Smoothie.
>
> **Lunch:** Try the Everyday Easy Salad with hemp seeds and sprouts.
>
> **Dinner:** Feast on Kale Avocado Salad with a Kick.
>
> **Snack:** Nibble on carrots and celery dipped in Zucchini Hummus.
>
> **End the day:** Sip at least 8 ounces warm lemon water.

Again, we recognize that you most likely associate with a little from each of these profiles and that your health challenges and food preferences are variable from season to season, day to day, and even hour to hour. These simple statements cannot completely define you because everyone's definition is a moving target. But picking your closest association enables you to have a clear point of entry. Remember, improvement in your health is not an all-or-nothing proposition. You should not be afraid of *subtlety*. Small changes can make a big difference and are far more sustainable for most people than a cold turkey approach.

In the following "Transition Days" chapter, we discuss those days between now and the first day of the cleanse that help ease you into the program. These days are a great way to dip your toe in the water, so to speak. But why wait until then? You can start now by *slowly* cutting out the items from the "Foods to Keep Off Your Plate" list in the next chapter. Drink water religiously, and begin introducing fresh fruit or green smoothies to your breakfast. Enjoy lots of salads and/or steamed veggies so the mainstays of your meals are vegetables. Think of the protein or the grain as a side dish. Begin to shift your perspective now as a sort of training for the cleanse.

And if you find yourself famished at any point, *eat.* Follow the guidelines of the program, and don't be afraid to turn your old notions on their head. It's okay to have a 4-ounce chicken breast as a snack after breakfast, especially if you're used to something a bit hardier than a smoothie. Begin to practice eating slowly and mindfully. Chew and really consciously taste your foods. Pay attention so you can catch yourself if you start shoveling it in. In a nutshell, *start thinking about your eating.*

A Word About Supplements

To supplement or to not supplement? It's a question we've wrestled with since the very beginnings of the Conscious Cleanse. And the answer, as you may suspect, is different depending on your individual preferences and goals.

To be clear: supplements are in no way required to complete a successful cleanse. You can get all the nutrients you need by eating a whole-food diet. That being said, many of our participants like to take supplements while cleansing. Some report that the before-meal ritual in and of itself helps them stay on track. Others feel they get more of a "full-blown cleanout" from supplementing.

If you do decide to take supplements, it's important to note that not all products are created equal. (For more information, as well as recommendations on brands we like best, visit consciouscleanse.com.)

A good colon cleanse supplement regimen contains an herbal blend, a high-quality fiber, and a toxin absorbent. The herbal blend draws out accumulated toxins from your body, supporting internal cleansing and healthy elimination. Look for a blend that contains minerals, enzymes, and healthy bacteria to nourish your bowels and digestive system.

The fiber bulks up your stool and works to remove toxins from your body. The most common is called psyllium fiber. Look for a supplement containing psyllium husks and seeds to get a blend of soluble and insoluble fiber.

And the toxin absorbent quickly absorbs and carries away old toxins as they're released into the bloodstream. This helps minimize the discomfort often associated with cleansing and detox.

Please remember that you don't need supplements to have amazing results with the Conscious Cleanse. In fact, a big green smoothie filled with dark leafy greens is loaded with fiber and produces a similar effect to any commercial fiber supplement *over time*. If you've been a meat eater for your entire life, love bread and pasta (gluten!), have a distended stomach, or have never cleansed before, you likely have build-up on your colon wall. To tackle this head on, you can supplement *or* commit to eating less meat during the cleanse. You may also want to commit to staying clear of the "food demons" even after you've finished the cleanse. As always, the choice is entirely yours.

The Importance of Food Combining

Brace yourself, because you're about to learn the world's best-kept secret to ongoing, effortless weight loss and management. Are you ready?

Eat in good, basic food combinations.

Of course, this simple statement carries some hefty and complex details, but we're going to look at its most basic and intuitive components. To begin, keep this formula in mind:

Waste = weight

Simply stated, if you're not eliminating after every meal, you're in some way storing waste, toxins, and fat in your tissues.

We've already talked a little about taking the strain off your digestive process to free up excess energy and how being conscious of the way basic food combinations work is crucial to that concept. We call these principles "easy in, easy out food combinations." At its most basic level, the theory is that we ideally eat foods that are easily and quickly digested and absorbed, with any leftover waste quickly processed and moved out of the body.

The faster the food is digested, the less waste it leaves behind. The less waste left behind, the easier the digestion process. When we eat in easy in, easy out food combinations, we free up significant energy in the body for deeper healing and cleansing. The results? Less weight, cellulite, inflammation, disease, headaches, acid reflux, gas, constipation, irritable bowel syndrome, and much more!

Okay, so let's look at the easy in, easy out food combining principles of the Conscious Cleanse. First, there are six basic food categories on the Conscious Cleanse you'll need to distinguish among:

1. Vegetables: any fresh vegetables, raw or lightly steamed
2. Animal protein: buffalo, lamb, fish, poultry, or wild game
3. Vegetable protein: nuts and seeds
4. Legumes and beans: lentils, black beans, adzuki beans, etc.
5. Nongluten grains: brown rice, quinoa, millet, buckwheat, etc.
6. Fresh fruit

In general, categories 2 through 5 mix well with category 1, but ideally they shouldn't be mixed with each other at the same meal. In other words, cooked or lightly steamed vegetables combine well with an animal protein, a vegetable protein, legumes, or a nongluten grain. Raw vegetables combine well with every category. Avoid mixing an animal protein and a grain in the same meal. Fresh fruit should always be enjoyed alone, with just a few minor exceptions (they combine well with dark leafy greens like in green smoothies, for example). The following table offers an at-a-glance guide.

Eat This ...	With This ...	But Don't Mix in Another of These ...
Vegetable	Animal protein	Vegetable protein, legumes and beans, nongluten grain
	Vegetable protein	Animal protein, legumes and beans, nongluten grain
	Legumes and beans	Animal protein, vegetable protein, nongluten grain
	Nongluten grain	Animal protein, vegetable protein, legumes and beans
Fruit	Leafy greens, cucumbers, celery	Vegetables, vegetable protein, animal protein, legumes and beans, nongluten grain

The main staple of the Conscious Cleanse is vegetables. So if you imagine a good-size plate, ideally two thirds of it should be filled with vegetables. The remaining third can be an animal protein, a vegetable protein, or a nongluten grain. So for a meal, choose a grain or a protein, but not both.

At your next meal, assuming at least about 3 hours have passed, feel free to switch your easy in, easy out food combination categories. For example, if you have a grain and vegetable for breakfast, it's completely acceptable to switch to a protein and vegetable for lunch.

Maybe this doesn't line up with what you're used to—the food pyramid you've heard so much about probably since elementary school or the My Plate variation released by the USDA in 2011. You aren't the only one who's been fooled into thinking these guidelines represent the "proper way" to eat for optimal nutrition.

What's Wrong with the Food Pyramid?

Many nutritionists and food research professionals agree that the USDA Food Pyramid is not only outdated given the current information available, but can actually be dangerous. The more updated My Plate version, although a huge improvement as far as a representation of a well-balanced diet, still misses some very important facets.

In his book *Eat, Drink and Be Healthy*, Harvard scientist Dr. Walter Millet calls out the myths of the traditional suggestions for balanced diet. Some of the facts he discusses that contradict the traditional food pyramid include the following:

Not all fat is bad. Saturated and trans fats are dangerous; polyunsaturated and monounsaturated fats like those found in raw nuts, fish, and olive oils are actually essential to heart health.

Not all complex carbohydrates are good. Choose nongluten whole grains versus even whole-grain bread, bagels, or pasta—enough said.

Not all sources of protein are the same. Red meat comes with saturated fats and cholesterol. Raw nuts? Not so much.

Dairy products are not essential to a balanced diet, right? Calcium comes readily—and is more easily absorbable—from sources like leafy greens, seeds, nuts, and beans.

Potatoes are not an important part of a standard diet. Don't confuse a potato for a vegetable. As a starch, potatoes can drastically increase your blood sugar levels.

A Note About Beans

Beans are technically both a complex carbohydrate and a protein and can be difficult to digest for some people, especially if they're not properly cooked. In general, it's best to soak and cook your beans from scratch (see Part 4 for suggestions) versus eating beans from the can. If you do use beans from the can, be sure to rinse them very well because they can contain a toxic residue. Also look for organic brands, like Eden Foods, which are packaged in custom cans with BPA-free lining.

If you have a lot of weight to lose or are dealing with any other digestive issues, you might consider minimizing or avoiding beans entirely during the cleanse. For food combining purposes, we treat beans and legumes like a protein to be mixed with veggies but not with grains.

The Convenience of Canned

There's no shame in using canned beans. They're much easier and faster to use, they're a healthy alternative, and often they're your only option. The downside of using canned beans is the increased likelihood of gas and BPA exposure. BPA stands for bisphenol A, a toxic chemical used to make some plastics and resins—like the resin lining used in canned foods to help preserve the contents. BPA has been linked to increased risk of breast and prostate cancers, infertility, obesity, and ADD/ADHD. If you use canned beans, rinse them several times before using. And never heat the beans in the water from the can—it will increase flatulence! Also, buy a BPA-free brand like Eden Organic beans.

A Note About Fresh Fruit

Ah, the myths of nutrition. Fruit is a perfectly healthy dessert, right? Sadly, that's not true. Especially after a cooked meal, fruit is actually a dessert best left in the fridge.

With a few exceptions, most fruit only takes about 30 minutes to digest, while most other foods take about 3 hours. When we eat fruit on top of food that needs longer in the stomach, a process of fermentation begins. The fermented fruit causes all sorts of nasty troubles, including gas and constipation, as well as bigger issues like toxic uptake and weight gain.

In the spirit of keeping things simple, consider eating your fresh fruit for breakfast, or as a snack by itself, and calling it a day.

A Note for the Plant Lover

If you're following the baseline plan and eating a mostly vegan, raw-food diet, you don't have to worry as much about proper food combining practices. It's still good to be aware, of course, but don't worry if a staple of your diet is, for example, apples and almond butter. When you eat lots of raw food, the live enzymes help your body digest the food so you're better able to tolerate it.

We know food combining can seem like a complex topic. It's important to know about it, but it's equally important not to obsess. Our goal with the Conscious Cleanse is to keep things as simple as possible and celebrate the accumulation of small improvements.

Experiment with the basic guidelines outlined in this section during your transition days and throughout the Conscious Cleanse. If, after a meal, you're not feeling gassy or bloated and you continue to eliminate regularly and effortlessly, you've most likely found a good food combination for you. Just listen to your body, stay curious, and remember your road map is yours alone.

Understanding Purification

During the Conscious Cleanse, you have two opportunities to experience the purification process. Purification is a 2-day practice designed to truly rest your digestive system. While the bulk of the Conscious Cleanse is very mild, subtle, and accessible, the purification days involve what may seem like a little more restriction on the surface (although on a deeper level, we believe it offers complete freedom). During these days, you'll basically stick to nourishing liquids and fresh fruits and vegetables exclusively.

We want to introduce this topic now so you can start to think about taking on the process. While it's completely optional, many of our participants find it to be a crucial component to deepening their experience.

Conscious Success: Savoring the Purification Process

Becky is an extremely active and healthy mother of three small children. She has known about her gluten sensitivity for several years and, with a few exceptions, avoids it completely. For her friends and family, Becky is the go-to gal for all things health-related.

Becky participated in the Conscious Cleanse as a way of giving back to herself for a change. Prior to the cleanse, Becky had been very busy working on a project, and in her hurried pace, she stopped listening to her body's cues. Prior to starting the cleanse, Becky's biggest complaint was her debilitating PMS. She had hoped to lose a few pounds and to get her coffee cravings under wraps, too.

"I LOVED the purification process," she relates. "I woke up after two days of veggies and fruits and felt like a million bucks. Day #1 I felt great, satiated and well all day. Day #2, I started my cycle at 5 A.M. But I only had cramps for about 15 minutes, and otherwise, I did not even notice it. That's huge for me. My moods were steady; I was not in pain; I pooped … it was great! I plan to drink a super green smoothie as my afternoon snack, or if I can manage to skip the afternoon eating, then to have it right after dinner to deal with my sweet tooth desires!"

Throughout the cleanse, Becky was able to reaffirm for herself the effects of sugar (even in the form of fruit!) on her moods and weight.

So what's the importance of purification? Purification helps us rest, heal, and lose excess weight. As you know, you spend approximately 3 or 4 hours and up to 80 percent of your body's energy digesting each meal. Freeing up that energy equates to turning over new cells and healing/detoxifying other organs like your kidneys, liver, and gallbladder. You'll rev up your metabolism, release toxins from the tissues, and burn stored fat.

Take It Easy

Purification happens during Days 6 and 7 and Days 13 and 14. Keep your schedule light during these days. This is a time for rest and rejuvenation. Don't plan a back-country ski trip or busy weekend. If you start the cleanse on a Monday, purification will fall over the weekends.

On a physical and emotional level, purification results in a feeling of being lighter and more energetic. The whites of your eyes get brighter, and your skin softens. On a deeper level, you may notice more mental clarity, more awareness, and easier decision-making. You may feel more open and more in tune with your body and your surroundings. We'd say that's worth it.

Rethinking Your Shopping Cart

You cannot change your destination overnight. But you can change your direction overnight.

—Jim Rohn

It's time to start thinking specifically about what you're going to eat during your 2-week cleanse. As you begin to put together your shopping list—and it's important that you have a shopping list!—keep in mind what you've learned so far, and continue to focus on what you *do* get to eat.

Because you're breaking out of your comfort zone and old habits, the supermarket can suddenly seem overwhelming. Take a breath. Remember the first day of school? The first day at a new job? It's all good. You'll settle in. We promise.

Remember to keep it simple as you shift your perspective on grocery shopping. Almost all your time is going to be spent along the perimeter of the store, among the whole foods. Take your cart out of autopilot mode. Really make this a joyful part of the experience rather than something you need to "get through." Spend time really looking at all the produce available. Take your time. Notice the items you may never have paid attention to before. How might incorporating these into your meals help broaden your horizons? Practice with parsnips. Get creative with collards. You don't have to go far to expand your world.

Conscious Eating Guidelines: A Review

Before we jump into creating your shopping list, let's do a quick check of what we've discussed so far. Keeping these points in mind helps when you're standing in the market wondering what to put in your basket, or in your kitchen wondering what's for dinner.

Feel free to come back to this section any time you need a refresher.

The Basics

Eating the "Conscious Cleanse way" is quite simple, but when in doubt you can come back to these basics:

- Eat whole foods that exist in nature.
- Eat raw and living foods as much as possible.
- Eat in easy in, easy out food combinations.
- Eat "clean" foods.
- Eat when you're hungry.
- Eat foods you like, and be flexible.
- Keep it simple, and constantly experiment.

Amazing Changes

Remember, if you simply add more fruits and vegetables to your diet, you'll begin to see amazing changes in your body and your life.

Overview of a Typical Meal

Remember the baseline of the Conscious Cleanse eating plan is veggies, supplemented with either a protein or a nongluten grain. When in doubt, you can always turn back here to review.

- Eat 4 to 8 ounces animal or vegetable protein per meal *or* 1 or 2 cups cooked nongluten grain per meal. (Choose protein *or* grain, not both.)
- Eat *unlimited* raw or lightly steamed vegetables and fruits.
- Include 1 or 2 tablespoons healthy oil (olive, borage, flaxseed, hemp seed, and sesame and coconut when cooking) per meal
- Drink lots of water.

Easy in, Easy out Food Combining Overview

Remember, veggies are your baseline and can combine with protein or grains. Eat fruit alone and on an empty stomach.

Here are a few more basics to keep in mind:

- Proteins combine with veggies.
- Grains combine with veggies.
- Avoid combining proteins and grains in the same meal.
- Examples of vegetable proteins include beans, nuts, and seeds. (Choose beans *or* nuts/seeds, not both.)
- Try to eat more vegetables than fruits by a ratio of 3:1.

Foods to Keep Off Your Plate

These are the no-no foods you should keep off your plate during the cleanse. Rather than "avoiding" these foods, make a conscious choice to keep them off your plate. Making that choice is making a good decision for you.

- Alcohol
- Caffeine
- Chocolate
- Corn
- Dairy (cheese, yogurt, milk, whey protein, and butter)
- Eggs
- Grapefruit
- Nightshades (potatoes, tomatoes, eggplants, and peppers)
- Oranges
- Peanuts
- Shellfish
- Soy (tamari, tofu, tempeh, miso, and edamame)
- Squash and sweet potatoes
- Strawberries
- Sugar
- Wheat and gluten products
- Yeast (and yeasted products like brewer's yeast, kombucha, and some fermented foods)

Steer Clear of the Food Demons

For a list of wheat and gluten products to avoid, see the "Battling the Food Demons" section in the first chapter.

Commit, and Be Kind to Yourself

Throughout the cleanse, remember to breathe deeply. Focus on how you're feeling, and stay positive! Respectfully disagree with the voice that says, *I can't do this, I don't understand, It's too hard,* or *I can't take this all in.* Know that there is no such thing as perfect.

Practice the art of non-negotiable commitment to your goal and nonjudgmental forgiveness of yourself. Remember that stress and guilt are toxins, too, and let them go.

Remind yourself that the only thing that matters is today. Remind yourself that you are strong. Make your choices from that place of strength, and feel yourself get stronger by the moment. Know that you are unique, you are one of a kind, but you are not alone.

Commit to This!

99 percent is a b---h. 100 percent is a breeze.

—Jack Canfield

Tips for Conscious Shopping

It's strange how a simple trip to the grocery or health food store can suddenly seem daunting, isn't it? Embrace that, but don't sweat it! Remember that any time you try something new, you're bound to experience some anxiety or excitement. With that in mind, we'd like to share some basic guidelines that will help you take on your new way of looking at the grocery aisles.

First, fill your grocery cart with as many fresh vegetables and fruits as possible. Represent all the colors of the rainbow in your food choices. Also, shop the perimeter of the store, only going "inside" for things like spices, nut butters, nut milks, and oils. You'll notice that all the "good stuff" is on the periphery: fresh produce, organic meats, wild fish, etc.

Buy your nongluten grains, raw nuts, and seeds in the bulk section. These items are often fresher, there's less packaging to recycle, and you'll save money. Shop for as many "package-free" foods as possible.

Shop for local, seasonal foods as much as possible. Check out produce from your local farm stand or farmer's market if they're available. You can't beat the quality or the shopping experience. Buy organic whenever possible to reduce your exposure to toxins, and familiarize yourself with the "Dirty Dozen" list. And be sure to buy more produce than you think you'll need. Because you'll need it.

The Dirty Dozen

It's important to reduce your exposure to toxins wherever possible. Eating pesticide-, herbicide-, and generally chemical-free organic whole foods is the most basic way to do this. The Environmental Working Group (EWG; ewg.org) annually ranks the Dirty Dozen—the foods that tested with the highest levels of toxic pesticide residue. Here's the current list as of this writing: apples (including apple juice and applesauce), celery, strawberries, peaches, spinach, imported nectarines, imported grapes (including raisins), sweet bell peppers, potatoes, blueberries, lettuce, and kale/collard greens (tie). Opt for organics of these foods to reduce your exposure to harmful chemicals. EWG also makes a great mobile app with the current Dirty Dozen and Clean Fifteen lists.

Frozen vegetables and fruits are a fine alternative to fresh, especially if you live in a cold climate where fresh vegetables and fruits aren't available. Canned and jarred versions often contain sugars, preservatives, or additives. If you must buy them, be sure you read the label closely.

Don't be afraid to ask for help. Don't know where something is? Don't know *what* something is? Particularly in health food stores, the folks working the floor are often highly knowledgeable and willing to answer questions.

The Conscious Cleanse Shopping List

We've given you lots of great ideas already, but let's take it one step further. In this section, we've included a list of great food to stock up on during the Conscious Cleanse. We suggest having an idea of the specific meals you plan on preparing (and the snacks you might enjoy). Then ensure you have what you need for those times and supplement with other items off this list. Most importantly, have fun!

Nonstarchy fresh vegetables:

- ☐ Artichokes
- ☐ Asparagus
- ☐ Avocados
- ☐ Beets
- ☐ Bell peppers (red, orange, or green)
- ☐ Bok choy
- ☐ Broccoli
- ☐ Brussels sprouts
- ☐ Cabbage
- ☐ Carrots
- ☐ Cauliflower
- ☐ Celery
- ☐ Cucumbers
- ☐ Green beans
- ☐ Green onions
- ☐ Leeks
- ☐ Okra
- ☐ Onions
- ☐ Parsnips
- ☐ Radishes
- ☐ Shallots
- ☐ Snow peas
- ☐ Sprouts (all varieties)
- ☐ Wild mushrooms
- ☐ Zucchini

Dark leafy greens:

- ☐ Arugula
- ☐ Beet greens
- ☐ Collard greens
- ☐ Dandelion greens
- ☐ Kale
- ☐ Romaine lettuce
- ☐ Spinach
- ☐ Swiss or rainbow chard

Fresh herbs:

- ☐ Basil
- ☐ Chives
- ☐ Cilantro
- ☐ Dill
- ☐ Fennel
- ☐ Garlic
- ☐ Gingerroot
- ☐ Mint
- ☐ Oregano
- ☐ Parsley
- ☐ Rosemary
- ☐ Sage
- ☐ Thyme
- ☐ Watercress

Fresh fruit:

- ☐ Apples
- ☐ Apricots
- ☐ Bananas
- ☐ Blackberries
- ☐ Blueberries
- ☐ Cantaloupe
- ☐ Cherries
- ☐ Coconut
- ☐ Grapes
- ☐ Honeydew
- ☐ Kiwifruit
- ☐ Lemons
- ☐ Limes
- ☐ Mangoes
- ☐ Nectarines
- ☐ Papayas
- ☐ Peaches
- ☐ Pears
- ☐ Pineapples
- ☐ Plums
- ☐ Raspberries
- ☐ Watermelon

Vinegars:

- ☐ Apple cider vinegar
- ☐ Balsamic vinegar
- ☐ Brown rice vinegar
- ☐ Ume plum vinegar

Oils:

- ☐ Borage oil
- ☐ Coconut oil
- ☐ Flaxseed oil
- ☐ Hemp seed oil
- ☐ Olive oil
- ☐ Sesame oil (not toasted)

Raw nuts and seeds:

- ☐ Almonds
- ☐ Brazil nuts
- ☐ Chia seeds
- ☐ Flaxseeds
- ☐ Hazelnuts
- ☐ Hemp seeds
- ☐ Macadamia nuts
- ☐ Pecans
- ☐ Pine nuts
- ☐ Poppy seeds
- ☐ Pumpkin seeds
- ☐ Sesame seeds
- ☐ Sunflower seeds
- ☐ Walnuts

Nut and seed butters:

- ☐ Tahini
- ☐ Raw almond butter
- ☐ Raw cashew butter
- ☐ Raw walnut butter

Spices and sweeteners:

- ☐ Allspice
- ☐ Bay leaves
- ☐ Cayenne
- ☐ Cinnamon
- ☐ Cloves
- ☐ Coriander
- ☐ Cumin
- ☐ Curry
- ☐ Curry paste
- ☐ Herbamare
- ☐ Herbs de Provence
- ☐ Himalayan crystal salt or Celtic Sea salt
- ☐ Honey (used sparingly)
- ☐ Oregano
- ☐ Paprika
- ☐ Pepper, black or white
- ☐ Pure maple syrup (used sparingly)
- ☐ Rosemary
- ☐ Stevia
- ☐ Turmeric
- ☐ Vanilla extract

Nongluten grains and seeds:

- ☐ Amaranth
- ☐ Black rice
- ☐ Brown rice
- ☐ Buckwheat
- ☐ Millet
- ☐ Quinoa
- ☐ Wild rice

Legumes:

- ☐ Adzuki beans
- ☐ Black beans
- ☐ Black-eyed peas
- ☐ Chickpeas (garbanzo beans)
- ☐ Lentils
- ☐ Split peas

Animal protein:

- ☐ Buffalo or bison
- ☐ Cold water fish (wild salmon, cod, halibut, and sole)
- ☐ Free-range chicken, turkey, and duck
- ☐ Lamb
- ☐ Wild game (venison, quail, pheasant, and rabbit)

Superfoods:

- ☐ Açai (powder or frozen, sugar free)
- ☐ Blue-green algae
- ☐ Goji berries
- ☐ Hemp seeds
- ☐ Maca
- ☐ Medicinal mushrooms
- ☐ Sea vegetables
- ☐ Spirulina

Other foods:

- ☐ Chicken or vegetable stock
- ☐ Chickpea miso
- ☐ Dijon mustard (no sugar)
- ☐ Fresh olives in water
- ☐ Fresh sauerkraut

Beverages:

- ☐ Coconut water
- ☐ Herbal teas and infusions
- ☐ Nut milks (almond, coconut, hazelnut, hemp, and Brazil nut; best if prepared fresh)

When you're shopping, knowing what brand to look for can be a big help, especially when you're trying something new. Here are some brands we like and trust:

Artisana's: tahini and cashew butter

Bragg's: apple cider vinegar

Bubbie's: sauerkraut

Eden Foods: beans, Ume plum vinegar, and seaweed gomasio

Frontier Natural Products Co-Op: herbs for herbal infusions, spices, and loose tea

Go Raw: flaxseed crackers

Kaia Foods: kale chips

Maranatha's: raw almond butter

Navitas Naturals: maca and açai powder

Pacific: organic almond milk, hemp milk, and chicken and vegetable broth

South River (southrivermiso.com): chickpea miso

Sweet Leaf: stevia

The Tea Spot: loose herbal teas

Zuké (esotericfoods.com): fermented foods

Fresh Almond Butter

You can buy freshly ground raw almond butter from some health food stores. Just be sure it's raw and not roasted.

Stocking Your Tool Kit

One of the most frequent questions we get from new participants is, "Will I have to spend all my time in the kitchen?" There's definitely some kitchen time required, but a little strategic planning can make meal preparation a relatively simple and unobtrusive task.

The most important tools you need are a sharp knife, cutting board, high-speed blender, to-go storage containers (we prefer glass ones), a cooler bag, and ice packs. You'll use these items every single day.

It's optional but helpful to have a food processor, possibly a juicer and nut milk bag (to make fresh nut milks, available online), but these are optional items. They're not required to have a successful cleanse.

Always always always prepare more food than you plan to eat at any given meal. You can pop the leftovers in the fridge for a snack or lunch the next day. It's so easy to make a salad for lunch tomorrow while you're prepping dinner for tonight. Just be sure to hold the dressing and add it the next day just before you're ready to eat it.

Make a big batch of salad dressing, your favorite "go-to" dip (like our Zucchini Hummus), and other yummy snacks (like our Joy Balls). Do this once a week (maybe on a Sunday evening?) so you'll be set when hunger strikes or when time doesn't allow for a ton of prep.

Likewise, make a stir-fry veggie grab bag. Chop up some broccoli, bok choy, celery, cabbage, onions, peppers, or any other veggies you like, and store in an airtight container. When you're ready to cook, all you do is grab and steam.

Make a raw salad veggie grab bag. Shred a few carrots, some parsnips, and some purple cabbage, and chop some celery. Toss together in an airtight container. Use for salads or wraps.

Produce Storage Tips

It helps to prep your vegetables and fresh fruit immediately after you get home from the grocery store and store them for quick and easy snacking. You're more apt to make good choices—fresh vegetables and fruits—when you have these ingredients cleaned, chopped, and ready to nibble on when your stomach rumbles.

To that end, here are some tips for successful produce prep and storage:

Apples   Store apples in a plastic bag in the refrigerator, ideally in the crisper section, away from strong-scented foods so they don't take on other flavors. Apples will keep for up to 10 days.

Avocados   Store at room temperature. Retain the pit, and store with any unused avocado to help keep avocado from turning brown. Avocados will keep for 1 day in the refrigerator this way.

Bananas   Store bananas at room temperature. To ripen green bananas, put them in a sealed plastic bag and set in a warm spot such as on top of the refrigerator. If you have overripe bananas, put them in the freezer to use in smoothies. Just peel them, pop them into a zipper-lock plastic bag, and freeze for later.

Broccoli   Wash and cut as soon as you get home from the grocery store. Store broccoli in a glass container for up to 3 days.

Cabbage   A whole head of cabbage lasts at least a week when stored in a plastic bag in the refrigerator's humid vegetable bin. Consume savoy and napa cabbage within 3 or 4 days. We like to shred purple cabbage immediately after shopping and store in a glass container in the refrigerator to be used for easy (and colorful) salad topping.

Carrots   Before storing carrots, remove their green tops, wash the carrots, and put them in a plastic bag. Store in the coldest part of the refrigerator with the highest humidity, and they'll last several months. You can also cut large carrots into easy-to-grab sticks and refrigerate them in a glass container with a small amount of water to keep them crisp for up to 5 days. These make for a great quick snack.

Cauliflower   Place cauliflower in a plastic bag and store it in your refrigerator crisper. When stored properly, cauliflower will last up to 5 days; however, it's best when eaten within 3 days.

Celery   To store celery, trim the base and remove any damaged or bruised leaves or ribs. Rinse, place in a plastic bag, and keep in the refrigerator's humid vegetable bin for about 2 weeks. Alternatively, chop into celery sticks and refrigerate in a glass container with a small amount of water for up to 7 days.

Chard   Refrigerate chard in plastic wrap for 2 or 3 days. Wash and chop only as needed.

Cilantro   Wash and dry thoroughly, and refrigerate in an airtight container with a loosely wrapped paper towel around it. Cilantro will keep for up to 5 days like this.

Collards   Wrap unwashed greens in damp paper towels, and refrigerate in a plastic bag in the crisper section for up to 5 days.

Grapes   Before storing, remove any spoiled or broken grapes. When refrigerated, they should keep for up to a week. During storage period, continue to remove spoiled fruit. Grapes can also be frozen for a yummy, cool, and sweet treat. They'll last up to 3 months this way. Be sure to remove the grapes from the vine before freezing.

Green beans   Place whole, unsnapped green beans in a perforated plastic bag or paper bag, and store them in the refrigerator crisper for up to 5 days. Wash and snap just before use.

Kale   Wash and de-stem kale, refrigerate in a plastic bag in the crisper section, or store directly in the salad spinner for up to 5 days. Be sure kale is fully dried before you store it.

Kiwifruit   Very firm kiwifruit (or kiwi) can stay in the refrigerator for up to 6 months. To ripen kiwis, keep them at room temperature away from heat or direct sunlight for up to a week. Store ripe kiwis away from other fruits. Ripe kiwis keep for about 1 or 2 weeks.

Lettuce   Refrigerate unwashed leaves in a plastic bag in the vegetable drawer for up to 5 days. Do not store lettuce with melons, apples, pears, or other ethylene gas–emitting fruits because they'll turn the lettuce brown.

Mangoes   Leave unripe mangoes at a cool room temperature for a few days to soften and sweeten. Very warm temperatures can cause an off flavor to develop. Place in a paper bag to speed ripening. Ripe mangoes are best kept in the refrigerator for 2 or 3 days.

Melons   Ripe whole or cut melons, wrapped tightly in plastic, can be stored in the refrigerator for about 3 days. Leave the seeds inside a cut melon until you're ready to eat it to help keep the melon moist. Store at room temperature to ripen.

Onions   Store whole, uncut onions in a dry and dark, well-ventilated place, not in the refrigerator. Once cut, store in an airtight container in the refrigerator for up to 5 days.

Parsley   Wash and dry thoroughly and store in an airtight container loosely wrapped in a paper towel. Parsley will keep for up to 5 days like this.

Pears   Store at room temperature. To ripen pears, store them in a sealed plastic bag with a couple ripe bananas at room temperature. Once the pear is ripe, refrigerate it until you're ready to eat it.

Spinach   Immediately wash spinach, trim the stems, and remove any blemished leaves. Repeat if necessary until you're sure all the grit and dirt has been removed. Spin dry in a salad spinner or allow to drain well. Refrigerate in the humid crisper section in a clean plastic bag very loosely wrapped with paper towels. Spinach will only last 2 or 3 days, so plan on eating it right away.

Go Green

If you want to go a bit greener, swap the plastic bags for cloth storage bags or cotton dishtowels to store your veggies!

Transition Days

Adopt the pace of nature: her secret is patience.

—Ralph Waldo Emerson

Imagine a pool full of cool, clear water on a hot summer day. There are two ways in: the first is taking a deep breath, closing your eyes, and hurtling yourself at the water; the second is slowly coming down the stairs, one step at a time, gradually acclimating. The end result is the same: you're fully submerged and happy to be there. In the parlance of pool-goers, "It's great, once you're in."

As you may have gathered, the Conscious Cleanse is the pool in this analogy. You can get in any way you want. Ultimately your body will adjust, and you'll feel comfortable and refreshed (so much so, you probably won't want to get out!). But here's the thing: because the Conscious Cleanse is about relishing the *experience* and practicing *mindfulness*, we're going to suggest that, even if you're a cannon-baller by nature, you try the coming-down-the-stairs approach, rather than just jumping in.

Slow change—change that occurs gradually—makes sustainable, long-lasting change. Over the years, many of our participants have commented that their changes were so gradual, they barely missed some of the things they'd given up. That's part of the point. The cleanse isn't about bulling your way through 2 weeks with sheer willpower; it's about setting the stage for true foundational change. By weaning yourself off your old habits and addictions slowly and methodically—rather than diving headlong into a cold-water shocking of the system—you'll get a clearer sense of where you're going, of how those habits and addictions were affecting you, as you let go of each one *consciously* through a process called "crowding out."

About Crowding Out

Rather than focus on what you *can't* have (restriction), shift your focus to the abundance of good, healthy foods you *can* have. Adding those to your diet "crowds out" the other stuff. What you'll soon discover is that by filling your focus with a bounty of whole foods, you push aside the foods you once craved. Eventually, you'll no longer need to force yourself away from them.

To that end, we suggest giving yourself a 5-day transition period as you move into your cleanse. We've designed these 5 days to be your measured entrance into the program, each day building on the previous one, so that on your official Day 1, you'll find that you're already comfortably submerged. And trust us, it is *great* once you're in.

Transition Day 1: Add More Vegetables and Fruits

Before we dive into all the things we *aren't* going to eat for the next several weeks, it's important to turn our attention to the abundance of foods we *do* get to eat and explore, perhaps for the first time. Quite simply, eat more vegetables and fruits.

Have a big green salad with your lunch and an apple for a snack. Eat more fresh vegetables and fruits than you did yesterday. Fresh foods like asparagus, beets, radishes, celery, cucumbers, carrots, spinach, bananas, pears, blueberries, grapes, kiwifruit, peas, broccoli, cauliflower—you get the idea. Fill your plate with color!

Transition Day 2: Eliminate Sugary Foods and Alcohol

Ah sugar, you addictive little devil! That fleeting rush of happy energy you offer—we get why you're such a hard habit to break. But the results are in: sugar is making us sick. And once you start looking for it, you'll find it's hidden in nearly everything.

On Day 2 of your transition, we ask you to start looking at where sugar may be lurking in your current diet. Eliminate *all* forms of processed sugar: cereals, cookies, cupcakes, pastries, candy, soda (including diet soda), fruit juice (that includes Naked and Odwalla-type juices), kombucha, flavored yogurt, artificial sweeteners (like Equal and Splenda), and high-fructose corn syrup. Also say a temporary good-bye to wine, liquor, beer, and other forms of alcohol, which likewise serve to spike your blood sugar levels and interfere with your body's ability to absorb nutrients.

Transition off processed sugary snacks by using *small amounts* (1 teaspoon in 1 cup of tea, for example) of natural sweeteners like honey, maple syrup, agave, or stevia. Have a small handful of dried fruit like raisins, dried cranberries, or dried mango to soothe the sugary beast, should she rear her ugly head (*during transition only!*). Eat sweet vegetables like roasted carrots and beets. Enjoy a colorful fruit salad made from low-glycemic fruits like blueberries, blackberries, and raspberries. These foods are naturally sweet and give you the energy your body craves.

The Glycemic Index

The glycemic index (GI) rates carbs on a scale of 0 to 100 based on how they affect blood sugar. Foods with a high GI (over 70 percent) tend to spike the blood sugar. Low-GI (under 55 percent) foods produce gradual increases in blood sugar and have a better effect on your overall health. High-GI foods include watermelon (80), baked white potatoes (98), and whole-wheat bread (78). Low-GI foods include apples (28), peaches (28), lentils (26), and rye bread (50). If you're sugar sensitive, opt for only low-GI fruits in your smoothies and as snacks. For more information and a comprehensive food search option, visit glycemicindex.com/foodSearch.php.

Transition Day 3: Eliminate or Reduce Your Caffeine Intake

We know, we know. Most people would rather cut off their right arm than give up their morning latté. Taking on this beast is often one of the biggest challenges our participants face. For an addictive diuretic stimulant, coffee sure must have a good marketing department. What we hear, all the time, is this: "I *like* my coffee. I *look forward* to my coffee."

First of all, don't tell yourself you're giving it up forever. Tell yourself you're taking a break or doing an experiment. Then take it slow. If you're a 6-cups-a-day kind of person, try cutting back to a couple cups. Tomorrow, go for the half caf (half caffeine/half decaf). The next day, transition to black tea, then to green tea, and then to herbal tea or warm lemon water … and there you are!

Also remember that each day is building on the next, so be sure to steer clear of adding sugar. After tomorrow, avoid dairy creamers. You may actually find this is a big help in letting go of your favorite hot beverage for a few weeks.

Once off the rocket fuel, you may find it's important to replace your morning ritual. We love warm water with lemon or a nutrient-rich herbal infusion. The warm lemon water gets things moving, if you know what we mean! (See Part 4.)

My Aching Head

As you come off caffeine, you may very well encounter some significant headaches. That's detox, friends! It'll pass, but in the meantime, try drinking a green juice or smoothie to feed your body with vital nutrients and minerals. Try to avoid taking the easy route of popping an Advil, if at all possible.

Get ready to be delightfully surprised at how much more energy you have when you're not all hyped up on stimulants. It takes a few days, but it's amazing when you realize for the first time in a long time, you're no longer dependent on a drug to help get you going in the morning or to keep you going through the afternoon. It's liberating in a way you can't describe until you've experienced it. Your body is a wonder machine.

Conscious Success Story: Kicking Caffeine

Kim had never done a cleanse before, and she was nervous going in. She had a history of almost nightly nightmares for more than 5 years, and it affected her ability to get true rest. She was an avid coffee drinker and was "dreading the thought of having to give up caffeine for the cleanse." She told us she imagined it would be the first thing she would "reward herself" with after completing her program.

Upon starting the cleanse, however, she found that her nightmares stopped completely. As she describes it, "I was waking up feeling more energized than I did after a cup of coffee, and without experiencing my usual afternoon crash."

By the end of her cleanse, she found that her physical and emotional cravings for coffee were gone. "So many other areas of my life benefited from the cleanse," she explains. "My stress level and management, my overall mood and energy level, and even the way I see myself. I just didn't need the coffee anymore."

She goes on, "I feel beautiful from the inside out and have gotten many compliments in the last month about how 'radiant' I look. I am so happy I worked up the courage to do the cleanse and had no idea how many other benefits it would have besides getting rid of my nightmares. Not only have I not had a nightmare since I did the Conscious Cleanse, but I have never slept or felt better in my life!"

Transition Day 4: Eliminate Dairy, Eggs, and Soy

As we discussed in the section on food demons, you are not absorbing as much calcium as you may think (or have been brainwashed to believe) from pasteurized dairy products like milk and cheese, and in fact, these products can wreak havoc on your digestive system. And while eggs may be an excellent source of protein (and omega-3 fatty acids), they also are among the top allergens in our country. Soy arguably has some very positive qualities, too, but it's also one of the more genetically modified foods of our time, and that processed, fake soy "meat" is among the most mucus-forming foods on the planet.

If you're thinking, *I can't live without (fill in the blank)*, you'll likely benefit the most from eliminating these foods from your diet. All too often, we find that the foods we eat regularly—the ones we say we're "addicted" to—are the very foods to which we develop sensitivities.

On the Conscious Cleanse, we're going to avoid all dairy, including milk, cheese, butter, whey protein, yogurt, sour cream, cream cheese, and, yes, even ice cream. Luckily, there are a slew of milk alternatives now widely available. Transition by trying unsweetened (that means sugar-free) almond milk, hemp milk, coconut milk, or hazelnut milk. Eat hot brown rice porridge for breakfast instead of eggs and toast. Have a handful of almonds instead of a slice of cheese for a snack. Enjoy an appetizer of hummus and raw veggies instead of cheese and crackers.

Some faux cheeses can act as good "cross-over" foods, but if you can help yourself, don't go there. Many of these contain soy or whey. Focus on eating "real food," and you'll be set up for success.

Transition Day 5: Eliminate Gluten

Yeah, we know it's the latest craze (you even can order off the gluten-free menu at McDonald's!), but there really is a difference between the concept of avoiding gluten and, say, the low-carb phenomenon. Gluten, the protein found in wheat, barley, and rye, turns into a gluey paste in your system, with the potential for causing inflammation, disease, and weight gain. And like sugar and corn, it seems to be *everywhere*. There's a good chance that if you have gluten sensitivities, you don't even know it yet, explains Dr. Mark Hyman, author of *The UltraMind Solution*.

So for this transition day, try taking a break from crackers, bread, bagels, pasta, cereal, and other packaged or processed foods. Be fierce with yourself. Don't fall into the "just a little won't make a difference" trap.

A good transition option is to move to nongluten options like brown rice and quinoa. If you can't live without pasta, try (*during transition days only!*) rice noodles. You can also try quinoa pasta. There are also plenty of rice crackers out there. Be sure to look for a "gluten-free" stamp on the label. As you move into the cleanse, work to cut out all processed foods.

Remember, many gluten-free foods (like gluten-free bread) have lots of other ingredients like dairy, sugar, eggs, and soy. You've already eliminated these foods, so no need to put them back in! "Gluten free" does not necessarily equal "healthy."

Dealing with Transition Day Cravings

You might have cravings on your transition days. It's very likely, in fact. But you can successfully deal with them.

Research shows that cravings only last for 3 to 5 minutes. You may argue—we know we did!—whether this is true. Of course, for many of us, the catch is that they sometimes seem to come back every 3 to 5 minutes as well! If this is your experience, we have some tips that might help:

- Reach for a "healthy" alternative. And no, this does not include "gluten-free cookies." Opt for a small amount of dried fruit, cacao, or maybe even some dark chocolate (more than 70 percent cocoa).
- Have a dried date filled with some raw almond butter.
- Make Raw Brownies (see Part 4).
- Make a sweet smoothie like the Frothy Banana Milkshake (see Part 4).

- Try a healthy chocolate milkshake like Mint Madness (see Part 4).
- Brush and/or floss your teeth.
- Enjoy a sweet herbal tea with a small amount of stevia and almond milk.
- Leave the vicinity. Go for a walk, take a bath, or just get out of the kitchen or the living room or wherever else the snack attack generally occurs.

A Closing Note on Transition

Transition is a time to be gentle. Take it slowly and know that your best is good enough. Once you officially begin Day 1 of the Conscious Cleanse, you'll feel well prepared, less anxious. You'll have worked out some of the kinks for yourself already, mellowed the curve on the various effects of detoxification.

Eliminating comfort foods and drinks that we have grown to lean on every day can be a scary thing. It can be like taking away a baby's pacifier. You may want to kick and scream for the first few days, but your "new normal" will move you forward surprisingly quickly. So again, trust the process, and know that each day will only get better.

Setting Your Intention

Think of your intention as your mission statement for the Conscious Cleanse. This is truly your North Star. If the going gets rough, this is the goal or mission you'll come back to. Your intention should inspire you, regardless of how big or small it may seem, and enable you to take on each day's challenges.

When setting your intention, as we'll ask you to do in a minute, think big. Go beyond the surface. You want to lose weight? Great. But go deeper than that. Why do you want to lose weight? Think about what you really want for your life—your deepest desires. Then ask yourself, *Is there something behind that desire? Why do I want that for myself?* Once you've gone as far as you can go, you have found your intention. For example, you may truly feel that if you just lost some weight, everything would change. But at second glance, you realize what you really want is self-acceptance or joy.

Conscious Success Story: Setting Your Intention

Paulina joined the Conscious Cleanse because she was tired, overworked, and feeling sluggish. Her initial intention for the cleanse was simply to gain more energy. She was hoping to break her coffee addiction and stop eating late at night. She worked long hours at a restaurant, so this was a worthy—yet lofty—goal.

As Paulina contemplated each question in this chapter's "In Your Journal" section, she peeled back the layers of her superficial desires, discovering that what she really needed to do was leave her job! She also decided she was ready to finally quit smoking. These two monumental decisions led her to follow a life-long dream of going to a yoga training retreat in Bali.

As Paulina allowed herself to really feel what she wanted, on a soul level, she discovered a deeper place in herself. She declared her intention to create "clarity" in her life. And you know what? Paulina got her clarity—and then some.

Along the way, she also discovered courage and self-love. Paulina tells us she continues to have a green smoothie a day, is more in tune with what her body does and doesn't need, and is now on the path to truly determining her life's purpose. What started out as an intention to have more energy and to eat healthier turned out to put in motion the wheels for a completely life-changing process.

Of course, finding a deeper intention doesn't mean you need to revamp your entire life! A deep intention means something different for everyone, and no one can figure out your intention but you. Think about setting your intention as a contemplation on the reason you're here.

Deep, we know. But you're about to embark on a deep experience, so make the most of it! Stop and focus on this before moving forward. When it comes to your health, what is the *most* you can have? Losing weight? That's just the tip of the iceberg. You are so much more than the size of your thighs. Dream like a child. Everything is possible.

In Your Journal

Before you go any further, we ask that you answer the questions on this page. Don't just think about your answers; write them down in your journal. Then read over your answers and really consider them. Your answers will guide you to your intention. As you move into the Conscious Cleanse, think about this intention each morning and in the moments before you put something in your mouth. Ask yourself, *Why am I eating this?* You should be able to answer that question with your intention.

So grab a pen, and start writing the answers to these questions:

> What do you really want in your life?
>
> When you realize or achieve your goal, what will that give you?
>
> And what will *that* give you?
>
> What will *that* give you?
>
> And what will *that* give you?

Keep going like this until you feel you've hit on *the* goal, *the* intention, *the* ultimate success.

> My intention for the next 2 weeks of the Conscious Cleanse is

_____.

The Conscious Contract

There is no partial commitment to this program—or really, if you think about it, anything in life. You are either committed or you're not committed. It's that simple. You choose or do not choose. The Conscious Cleanse is not an all-or-nothing proposition, but the decision to be committed to this process has to be 100 percent.

Think of an Olympic athlete. When she practices, she practices to win. She knows she can't control the outcome, but she can control how invested she is in the game. What we know is that being partially committed—playing half out—is not possible.

Remember this is not about perfection. It's about having a bad day and picking yourself up with love. It's remembering that tomorrow is a new day. Regardless of your slip-ups, you don't check out, you don't quit, and you don't overburden yourself with guilt or self-loathing. You might want to reread that last sentence.

You stay. Regardless of how "good" you've been, you stay. You show up tomorrow because you know each day is different. And this is life. You're not committing to perfection. You're committing to your intention. The great

Earl Nightingale said, "Success is the daily progression of a worthy ideal." Commit to that kind of success. Isn't your life a worthy ideal?

Copy this page or download it from our website (consciouscleanse.com), and post it where you'll see it every day:

The Conscious Commitment

As a participant of the Conscious Cleanse, I promise ...

- To make healthy decisions to the best of my ability.
- To know when to be fierce with myself and when to be gentle.
- To celebrate my successes as well as my challenges.
- To be curious and to listen to my body.
- To recognize my journey as unique to me.
- To remember to laugh and trust that my best is good enough.
- To allow myself to heal physically, emotionally, and mentally.
- To love, honor, and appreciate myself just for showing up.

With love and acceptance,

_____

Your signature

_____

Date

Part 2

The Conscious Cleanse

Welcome to the Conscious Cleanse

The most powerful tool you have to transform your health and improve your mood, mind, and metabolism, is your fork.
—Dr. Mark Hyman, author of *The UltraMind Solution*

You did it! You're here! Committing to a process like this is often half the battle. So congratulations on a major first step! We know you may be feeling anxious or skeptical. Maybe you're worried you're going to be too hungry or you won't be able to maintain the cleanse for 2 weeks. Maybe you're just freaking out! There's no need to. Just relax and take it 1 day at a time.

One Day at a Time

Beginning a process like the Conscious Cleanse is like being at the starting line of a big race. The adrenaline begins to pump, you start to feel jittery, and maybe even a little doubt creeps in. And then the starting shot sounds! Before you know it, you're halfway through the first mile. As every good runner knows, the race is run 1 mile at a time. You focus on the mile you're running now because that's the only mile you can control.

Whatever it is that brought you here is in the past. Whatever lies ahead of you doesn't even exist. It's easy to overwhelm yourself by thinking about the past or the future. By focusing on the here and now, you'll find that things become surprisingly manageable.

So instead of getting overwhelmed and sabotaging your success, we want you to know it's all perfect just as it is. Your emotions are normal responses to beginning something new. So don't get stressed about being stressed or anxious about being anxious. Where your attention goes, your energy flows, so let go of that negative juju right now. Approach this process with a step-by-step, day-by-day plan, and know we'll be there at every mile marker, cheering you on.

Be Human

You cannot fail here. As we've said, there is no wagon, so there is no wagon to fall off of. The Conscious Cleanse is not about "doing it right" or being perfect. It's about being human.

We want you to spend each day noticing how certain foods feel in your body, but just as importantly, we want you to pay attention to your *emotional* reactions and triggers. Trust the process, and know that small changes make big differences over time, that every conscious decision you make is a stride forward, and that each mile of the race is an accomplishment in and of itself.

It's important for us to mention again that everyone's process is going to be different because everyone starts from a different place. You have your own habits and health concerns, your own goals, and your own distractions. You are your own best friend. Remind yourself that *you* always know what's best for you. During the Conscious Cleanse, you are your own best coach.

Your body has an inherent wisdom, and once you remove some of the noise—the sugar, the caffeine, the alcohol, and the other things that get in the way of being able to hear yourself—the messages start coming through loud and clear.

The Conscious Focus

Each day throughout the next 2 weeks, we invite you to read and consider the day's "Conscious Focus" section. These sections are designed to offer you daily nuggets of wisdom, inspiration, insight, and support—love notes from us, if you will, encouraging you to stick with the process and to thrive while doing so.

There's just no way around the fact that changing habits can be overwhelming. We've found that a single focal point can offer a place to return when the going gets tough. The "Conscious Focus" sections are meant to help you stay engaged and connected to the process.

Consider waking up a few minutes early, preparing yourself a cup of herbal tea, and sitting down to read the day's "Conscious Focus" section while free of distractions, before the rush and demands of the day. Don't just barrel through in a flurry to get a smoothie blended. Really immerse yourself in the experiment during your 2 weeks on the program, and give yourself the luxury of a few minutes of concentrated thought and reflection each day. It's amazing how rarely we make this simple time for ourselves, and even more amazing how revelatory it can be.

Become the Moment

If you pay attention at every moment, you form a new relationship to time. In some magical way, by slowing down, you become more efficient, productive, and energetic, focusing without distraction directly on the task in front of you. Not only do you become immersed in the moment, you become that moment.

—Dr. Michael Ray, author of *The Highest Goal*

Food, as we've said before, is never just about food. The "Conscious Focus" sections prompt you to take action every single day, to help your mind support your body along this transformative journey. These sections offer practical tips and tricks to fit the program into your daily life, but more than that, they help deepen your healing process by helping you concentrate on your own body-mind connection.

The Conscious Eating Meal Plan

By now you may be asking yourself, *So what* am *I going to eat for the next two weeks?* In the chapters that follow, we offer a sample meal plan for each day of the Conscious Cleanse. We give you the recipes for each of the items listed on the meal plans in Part 4 of the book.

We also give you a "baseline meal program" with suggestions for optional additions like animal protein or grains, as well as snack suggestions, for each day. It's important to note that these are *sample* meal plans. Feel free to follow them to the letter, or feel even freer to break from them, to experiment, to tweak your meals to suit your own tastes, particularly as the messages your body offers come more and more into focus.

Whether or not you choose to follow these meal plans, just remember that the foundation of the Conscious Cleanse is plant based. From that foundation, we offer suggestions for the "grain lover" and the "meat lover," as well as suggestions for satisfying your sweet tooth. If you're accustomed to eating a stick-to-your-ribs egg-and-toast kind of breakfast, for example, you may well start off with the meat- or grain-lover alternative. But for 2 weeks, think about adding meat or grains to your vegetables, as opposed to the other way around. Believe it or not, there's a significant mental shift involved in thinking of your meal as having some chicken with your broccoli as opposed to having some broccoli with your chicken, even if the plate looks the same in both cases.

Either way, this is not a plan about counting calories, points, or fat grams. When you eat mostly veggies and whole foods in their natural state, you'll quickly find that your body self-regulates, letting you know when you're naturally hungry—and when you're full. As you know, what should be a simple connection between mind and body is often muddied by modern diets, by chemically altered and processed foods, by added sodium, and by sugars that serve to trick us into eating more than our body actually wants. Well, no more!

A diet cannot be about willpower. Through this process, your body will reveal a wisdom to you. It will tell you what it needs for nourishment. So when you consider the following meal plans, don't get stuck on amounts or serving sizes. Put away your food scale. Eat when you're hungry, and stop when you're not. This is not, as our mothers used to say, the "clean your plate club." This is the "learn to listen to your body" club. Besides, leftovers make great snacks for later or meals for tomorrow. Likewise, if you finish what you've prepared and are still hungry, eat more. Simple, right?

Remember the Conscious Cleanse Basics

Before we move on to the first day of the cleanse, we want to lay it out again in a nutshell (raw and unsalted, of course) to minimize confusion:

Eat vegetables, ideally raw or lightly steamed. Go for it. Experiment. Get crazy. You can't overdo it on vegetables.

Add a protein or grain, but avoid adding both in the same meal. Eat 4 to 8 ounces animal or vegetable protein (nuts, seeds, or beans) per meal *or* eat 1 or 2 cups cooked nongluten grain (like brown rice or quinoa) per meal.

Focus on Plants

Remember, this is a plant-based diet with room for small amounts of poultry, fish, and wild game. We want to be very clear that the Conscious Cleanse is not an endorsement for eating unlimited amounts of meat. To get the results, focus on eating lots of vegetables.

Eat some fresh fruit, but try to keep your vegetable-to-fruit ratio as close to 3:1 as possible. Focus on low-glycemic fruits like pears, blueberries, apples, and peaches when you do enjoy fruit.

Rotate your food choices, and don't gorge on any one food. Consider multiple meals that don't include a meat or a grain.

Include 1 or 2 tablespoons healthy oil per meal. Healthy oils include olive oil, flaxseed, hemp seed, and borage. Steam or water stir-fry your vegetables, and drizzle the oil on top. Cook only with oils that can sustain high heats, like sesame and coconut oil.

Drink lots of water—at least half your body weight in ounces—every day. Start the day with 32 ounces warm filtered water with lemon, and drink purified water.

Remember that these guidelines are just that: guidelines. Start from where you are. Diet does not have to be all or nothing, and change does not have to be absolute.

Above all, be kind to yourself, listen to yourself, and trust yourself. No one knows you like you.

Day 1: A New Day

To live is an awfully big adventure.

—Peter Pan

Welcome to Day 1 of the Conscious Cleanse. Today is a new day. No matter how many cookies you've shoveled in your mouth or how much rocket fuel you've guzzled, today is a new beginning. We are committed to making the next 2 weeks a radically eye-opening and life-altering experience for you. Take it easy, and proceed with care. As long as you continue to add in more fresh fruits and vegetables, you will be on your way to many healing benefits.

Conscious Focus: Write in Your Daily Journal

Throughout the next 2 weeks (and hopefully for the rest of your life!) we want to help you turn your attention to the things you're doing well, to the abundance of foods you can eat, and to all your little successes by writing about them in your journal. After you've journaled for a few days, you can watch how quickly little successes become a book of successes!

Today's Action Step: Begin Your Mental Cleanse

One of the best ways to get into this mind frame is to do a "mental detox" every single day! This is a very powerful practice and something to do every single day throughout the Conscious Cleanse.

Set your alarm clock for 15 minutes earlier than normal. Get up, take care of basic business (go to the bathroom, brush your teeth, drink some water), and find a comfortable place to sit with your favorite pen and a journal. For the next 15 minutes, your task is to simply put pen to paper and write, uncensored, without stopping and without filtering, until 15 minutes is up.

In addition to morning journaling, we suggest end-of-day writing, and so at the end of each program day, we give you some cues to help you get going. Feel free to use these cues, or write your own thing. What you reflect on is much less important than the fact that you're taking the time to reflect.

This is a powerful and transformational practice. It's also an opportunity to do a "mental dump," to get all the negative self-talk, the worries, and the doubt out on paper. You'll be amazed at how differently the day goes.

Conscious Eating Meal Plan

Enjoy Day 1! You'll notice we offer several suggestions for each meal and your daily snacks. The recipes for all the suggestions are found in Part 4. Happy cleansing!

Begin the day:

> Drink 1 quart warm lemon water.

Lemon Water Ritual

One of our favorite cleanse rituals is drinking warm lemon water. As soon as you wake up, put on a teakettle of water. Then, cut a lemon in half and squeeze the juice of half of it into a quart-size mason jar. While your water warms, grab your journal and begin to write uncensored. When the water starts to steam (you don't have to bring it all the way to a boil), pour the warm water into the jar. Drink the entire quart before you eat or drink anything else. This lemon water gives you a burst of vitamin C, helps alkalize your blood, *and* helps gently stimulate your bowels so you can make your next stop the bathroom.

Breakfast:

> Drink 1 quart green smoothie of choice. Lost in all the choices? We suggest the Swiss Cinnamon Smoothie.

> Or if you're looking for something warm instead, try Raw Buckwheat Breakfast Porridge.

> If you're feeling foggy or need more protein, try a green smoothie and supplement your meal with 4 to 8 ounces chicken breast (or some other lean animal protein) about 1 or 2 hours later.

Lunch:

Eat a Super Big Easy Salad.

Need more protein? Add 4 to 8 ounces broiled salmon to any salad you like.

Today's snack ideas:

Enjoy some Kale Chips.

Or nosh a handful (about ⅓ cup) raw walnuts.

Carrot and celery sticks dipped in Zucchini Hummus, with an herbal infusion, also works.

Sensational Snacks

The snacks listed in this section are great for between breakfast and lunch or between lunch and dinner.

Dinner:

Cook some Vegetable Medley Stir-Fry, and enjoy with either 1 or 2 cups brown rice or 4 to 8 ounces chicken such as Basic Baked Chicken Breasts.

End the day:

Sip at least 8 ounces warm lemon water.

Ingredient of the Day: Kale

Kale is one of the best dark leafy greens out there—and no, it's not just a garnish. The most common types you'll see at the market are curly kale, dino (lacinato) kale, and purple kale. Kale is good for chronic inflammation (thanks to flavonoids, quercetin, and kaempserol), and it's a great source of calcium.

Eat organic kale as much as possible. It's one of the foods on the Dirty Dozen list. (See the whole list in the "Rethinking Your Shopping Cart" chapter, or better yet, download the mobile app from the Environmental Working Group.)

If you've ever tried making a salad out of raw kale, you may have run into some issues. It's hard, chewy, and dry—yuck. But wait, don't give up there. The secret to enjoying raw kale is the simple act of giving your kale a massage. *Oh boy*, you're thinking. *One day in and they already have me massaging vegetables.* But it's true, so give it a try by rubbing a touch of olive oil and sea salt on the leaves. *Voilà!* The kale is suddenly soft and delicious!

Another easy way to get your daily dose of this green love is to put it in a smoothie. If you're new to green smoothies, you might want to start slowly. Just add a little kale to your favorite recipe at first. Over time, you can ramp up so you're including a fistful of kale with your breakfast.

Need a great snack? Try our baked Kale Chips. Not only can they satisfy your taste buds with something salty and crunchy—they're packed with nutritious goodness.

Quick Tip: Pack Your Bag!

Staying on track with the Conscious Cleanse is all about planning ahead. Say it three times: *Plan ahead. Plan ahead. Plan ahead.* So before you venture out for the day or even for a quick errand, be sure you load up your "conscious snack pack." This is your ultimate key to success.

Here's what you need:

- A small cooler bag and ice pack
- Some airtight containers (We like glass.)
- Utensils and a napkin
- Quart-size glass mason jars or other large sealable cups for smoothies (You can buy a case of wide-mouth mason jars for less than a buck a piece at your local grocery store or online.)
- A large water bottle (We like LifeFactory glass bottles.)

And here's an example of what you can pack if you're going to be out over the course of several meals:

- A salad with lots of veggies and a lemon wedge
- A small container of homemade dressing
- A piece of fresh fruit like an apple or a pear
- A small baggie of raw nuts (about ⅓ cup)
- A (4- to 8-ounce) piece salmon

- 1 quart green smoothie
- A big bottle of purified water

We should note that there's a very good chance you won't need all this food in 1 day. The idea is to leave the house with more than enough in the event you're gone for the entire day or need to be out longer than expected. If you're running a quick errand, you might only pack a smoothie and a piece of fruit. Again, the point is to plan ahead so you don't get stuck looking for something cleanse-friendly at the local gas station convenience store.

In Your Journal

Today is Day 1 of journal writing! Put pen to paper and write, nonstop, uncensored, without filtering your thoughts, for 15 minutes.

Can't think of anything to write? Start with how you're feeling physically. Feeling light, tight, tired, or energized? How about emotionally? Are you grumpy, annoyed, excited, or worried? Don't think about it too much, just start writing!

Day 2:
Become a
Green Machine

You know who you are, but know not who you could be.
—William Shakespeare

Today is about being courageous. We know some of you reading this book are already full-blown health nuts, but let's face it: committing fully to a process like the Conscious Cleanse takes serious guts. It takes heart.

Regardless of your personal starting point, recognize when you're belittling yourself in any way right now and if you are, stand up and give yourself a giant hug of appreciation instead. Appreciate and love yourself for mustering the courage to pick up this book, for taking one step at a time. It's Day 2, and already, because of your courage, your eyes are brighter and your skin is beginning to glimmer. Take a look … the changes are already beginning to happen!

Don't forget to take that courage with you as you dive into your conscious focus of the day. Today we're going to convert you to a green guzzler!

Conscious Focus: Green Smoothies

Have you tried a green smoothie yet? Wow! This power-packed, nutrient-dense treat is one of the best ways to eat your greens! Greens are at the top of the whole foods world, chock-full of vitamins, enzymes, minerals, and trace minerals. They're also low in calories (not that we're counting calories, mind you!) and high in nutrients.

Did you know you can get more bio-available calcium from greens than from cow's milk? And rarely will you find a food with more fiber than dark leafy greens. The insoluble fiber in greens actually promotes regular bowel movements, so you're able to detoxify your system more efficiently.

We also love green smoothies because it can be a challenge to sit down and eat the quantity of greens found in a smoothie. When's the last time you ate a huge plate of chard? Never? Yeah, that's what we guessed. Kale, chard, spinach, collards, dandelion greens—it's all game here. And green smoothies are so tasty, even your kiddos will swallow them down and ask for more.

Sippable Smoothies

We've included some of our favorite smoothie recipes in Part 4. Feel free to try those or experiment with your own recipes. Once you start to get the hang of the general formula, you'll be tossing in whatever you have in the fridge. Have fun!

Today's Action Step: Experiment with Green Smoothies

Start today (and every day if you're up for it) with a green smoothie. It's a nutrient-dense way to begin your day. And it's a quick meal you can take on the go if you do have to run out the door. Forget the drive-thru, and grab a smoothie as your new fast-food meal.

Here are some simple secrets to making a green smoothie that rocks:

- 1 or 2 cups water (or try coconut water or almond milk occasionally)
- 1 or 2 large handfuls greens (or more if you like!)
- Fruit for sweetness

The goal is to load your smoothie with as many greens as you can. In the beginning, you might be more prone to the sweet smoothies filled with fruit and just a little of the green stuff. That's fine. Just go slowly and work your way up to savoring the delicious taste of chlorophyll (mostly greens and little to no fruit). In general, the darker the leafy green, the better, but as you're training your taste buds and detoxifying your system, start with the more mellow-tasting greens like romaine lettuce or spinach.

Chew On This

Be sure to chew your green smoothie a bit. Digestion starts in your mouth, and when you chew your food, you release important enzymes needed for digestion.

Conscious Eating Meal Plan

Welcome to delicious Day 2! Remember, these meal plans are suggestions; they are not hard-and-fast rules. As you move through the program, you'll gain the confidence and expertise to tailor each day to your specific needs and tastes. Of course, you can also feel free to stick to our examples if they work for you.

Begin the day:

Drink 1 quart warm lemon water.

Breakfast:

Drink 1 quart green smoothie of choice. Try the Green Goddess Smoothie. It's a great beginner smoothie.

Good Morning, Smoothie

I love the green smoothies! They actually get me eating in the morning, which is a huge problem for me. I feel my metabolism starting to rev up!

—Linda G., recent cleanse participant and green smoothie convert

Lunch:

Choose a large salad. We suggest the Kale Avocado Salad with a Kick. Want more protein? Add 4 to 8 ounces chicken left over from your dinner last night.

Today's snack ideas:

Nibble on 2 Protein-Packed Almond Butter Balls.
Handful of Kale Chips also works.
Or you can have your choice of green smoothie.

Dinner:

> Try a bowl of Curried Carrot Soup and a side salad of choice.
>
> If you're craving carbs, serve the soup over 1 cup brown rice or quinoa. (You also might want to make extra brown rice or quinoa for the rest of the week!)
>
> Or if you're craving protein, eat 4 to 8 ounces Ginger Broiled Salmon.

End the day:

> Sip at least 8 ounces warm lemon water.

Ingredient of the Day: Turmeric

Turmeric, one of the main ingredients found in curry, is not called the Golden Goddess of Herbs just because it tastes good! Research is now backing up what ancient cultures of India, Asia, and Africa have known for years: turmeric has some amazing healing properties, including its anti-inflammatory, anticancer, and antioxidant benefits. Turmeric can be used as a natural painkiller and helps relieve arthritis, muscle sprains, and swelling and pain from injuries. It also has amazing antibacterial benefits.

Mix 1 teaspoon turmeric with a bit of homemade applesauce for your daily dose.

Quick Tip: Dealing with Caffeine Withdrawal

Let's face it. Caffeine is a legal drug. It's a stimulant, and it's highly addictive. Assuming you've been weaning yourself off the hard stuff, let's talk about what to do if you're having caffeine withdrawal.

Sidestep your withdrawal by slowly weaning your way off caffeine as suggested in transition Day 3. Also, try some of the following suggestions when the symptoms—frequent headaches, fatigue, irritability, constipation, and lack of concentration—start to rear their ugly heads.

- Drink lots of water—and we mean *lots!*—to flush your system.
- Take a hot Epsom salt bath, being sure to dunk your head, especially if you're experiencing headaches.
- Rest or take a nap.
- Drink a green juice for a natural high.

- Drink herbal peppermint tea.
- Exercise to release natural endorphins.

Beware Painkillers

Avoid taking over-the-counter painkillers because some of these also contain caffeine and will just add to the toxic load you're working to minimize.

In Your Journal

What are you excited about as you start this process? What are you terrified of?

Day 3:
Shake Your
Groove Thang

If you are going through hell, keep going.

—Winston Churchill

Day 3. Hump day. Humps are tricky because they're kind of like hills, and because hills can sometimes feel challenging, we want to give you a big shout out today to remind you that you're amazing! You're doing it! And it doesn't matter if you think you're doing it "right" or not. What matters is that you're here, on the journey, reading this right now. It's okay if you're feeling lethargic or headachy, running to the bathroom to pee every 10 minutes, or dealing with intense sugar cravings. That's exactly where you should be.

So in the spirit of hills and challenges, think about the view from the top of the mountain. And think of how rejuvenated and alive you feel. You'll be there soon! Just keep going!

Conscious Focus: Move Your Body

We know we've been talking a lot about food. Well, now it's time to switch gears a bit and look at the whole-body picture. You want a balanced life, right? You want to thrive and feel like you have more than enough energy to get you through the day? Well, here it is: the human body thrives on movement.

Moving your body helps improve your mood, enhances your body confidence and body image, makes you feel revitalized, revs up your metabolism, curbs your cravings, improves your elimination, helps you lose weight, builds muscle, and increases your focus. When you "shake your groove thang," you get your lymphatic system pumping, which is one of the main ways your body takes out the trash. Try to break a sweat today. Those little beads of sweat help you release toxins through your skin.

Heal Thyself

According to Dr. Brian Clement of the Hippocrates Institute, the body heals eight times faster when you exercise regularly.

Here are some easy ways to get your body moving:

- Jump up and down or rebound on a mini trampoline.
- Go for a brisk walk. Be sure to swing your arms and breathe in the fresh air. Who cares if people give you funny looks?
- Put on your favorite music, and have a dance jam in the kitchen.
- Do some yoga or stretching.

Find a type of exercise that you love, that you have fun doing, and that doesn't require you to alter or rearrange your day too much. Can you take the stairs instead of the elevator? Get off the subway one stop early and walk the rest of the way? Jog in place? Do some push-ups? Take a hike with a friend? (The conversation alone will make your heart shine!) It doesn't matter how—just get your body moving!

Take note of how you feel before and after exercising. Initially, you might be exhausted. That's okay. Take it slowly, and don't blow your gasket your first day out. The more you move in ways that are fun and pleasurable to you, the more you'll start to recognize the new flow of feel-good endorphins. This is the best natural high around.

Today's Action Step: Get Shakin'!

Jump up right now and move your body. Enroll your best buddy, and go out for a walk. Put on some music, dance around your kitchen or office, or get yourself to yoga class. Do something you love! It's not about duration, calories burned, or pushing yourself past your edge.

Conscious Eating Meal Plan

As you get moving today, you may notice your appetite changes. It'll also be even more important to be sure you're drinking enough water, so keep it flowing! Remember to listen to your body and feed it what it needs.

Begin the day:

Drink 1 quart warm lemon water.

Breakfast:

Drink 1 quart green smoothie of choice. Try the Hearty Smoothie Love. It's a perfect, filling, beginner smoothie.

Lunch:

Eat a large salad. Try the Shredded Salad, and make extra for tomorrow's lunch!

Want more protein? Add 4 to 8 ounces Ginger Broiled Salmon from your dinner last night.

Today's snack ideas:

Choose some chilled sliced cucumber sprinkled with lime juice and sea salt.

A handful of nuts (about ⅓ cup), or any other leftovers should do nicely.

Dinner:

Enjoy Cauliflower Mashers with Mushroom Gravy and Marinated Greens.

Want more protein? Add some Wild West Buffalo—and make extra for lunch tomorrow!

End the day:

Sip at least 8 ounces warm lemon water.

Ingredient of the Day: Stevia

We all love something sweet, right? And here we are eliminating most of the sugar from your diet. We have some good news for you. Stevia is a perfect way to get your fix without the crash and burn effect of sugar.

Stevia is a zero-calorie herb from the Andes that's actually 200 to 300 times sweeter than sugar! This sugar substitute won't spike your blood sugar and in fact, doesn't contain any sugar at all! You can find stevia at your local grocery store or buy it online. Stevia comes in both powder and liquid form. Not all Stevia powders are created equal. Their taste, sweetness, aftertaste, and levels of refinement can affect whether or not you like it. Try a few brands to find the one you like the best. We love Donna Gates' Stevia Liquid Concentrate, available at bodyecology.com, and SweetLeaf, now available at most grocery stores.

Stevia can be used in tea, smoothies, salad dressings, desserts, breakfast cereals, homemade nut milks, and more.

Quick Tip: Dealing with Cravings

Cravings get a bad rep. They're the number-one complaint we hear about! We want to suggest that cravings aren't all bad. The problem is that cravings are generally running the show. So today we want to look at what your cravings are trying to tell you and what to do so they're no longer controlling your every move.

Love dark chocolate? Pastries? Candy? A beer or glass of wine at the end of the workday? How do you get your fix?

On the one hand, there's often a very physical reason for your body's cravings. When the sugar craving strikes, for example, it's often in response to your body's plea for more quick energy. Sugary snacks, dark chocolate, refined carbs—they all give you that quick burst of energy your body desperately needs. The problem is that when you always give in to your sugar craving, you are borrowing against the bank, so to speak, and reaffirming the crash and burn cycle. 'Round and 'round you go.

As you eliminate sugar from your diet, it's natural that your body is going to protest in some ways. You're now asking it to make its own energy, which it likely isn't used to doing.

Listen to your body, but be mindful not to give in to its every whim. As Julie always admits in our programs, "If I always listened to my body's wants and desires, I would be sitting on the beach drinking a margarita and smoking a cigarette." That's obviously not the body's innate wisdom speaking.

On the other side of the craving coin are the *emotional* factors. On a deeper level, it's good to take the magnifying glass to your cravings. When the craving hits, ask yourself, *What am I* really *craving?* Oftentimes, your cravings act as a mask for a larger issue going on in your life. Are you feeling unfulfilled at work? Is there a conversation you've been avoiding with a loved one? Is it time to change careers or jobs? Is there some void the craving of choice is filling?

Just by simply being in the inquiry with your cravings, things will start to surface. Take note. Get these thoughts and realizations on paper in your journal so they're no longer running the show. Be curious and forgiving, and don't forget to take deep breaths.

In Your Journal

What are you craving? What are you *really, really, really* craving? What are you struggling with? Food prep? Detox? Get it out on paper now. In the light of day, your problems suddenly seem more manageable, so get them out.

Day 4:
What Are You
Grateful For?

What lies behind us and what lies before us are tiny
matters compared to what lies within us.

—Ralph Waldo Emerson

Recall for a moment the last time you were in a funk. Were you depressed,
feeling alone, lost, or just out of it? And can you also remember the moment
when the lightbulb went on? When you had a stroke of inspiration, genius,
direction, and hope?

Well that, sweet friend, is what today is all about. It's about knowing and
feeling that just around the corner is a beautiful opening, a new chapter, the
dawning of your magnificence. So feel your stuff as it comes up with a bit of a
smirk today because now you know the truth. Bask in that today.

Conscious Focus: Cultivate an Attitude of Gratitude

Today is about gratitude. Some days it's hard to be grateful. Are you supposed to just ignore the fact that you're in a funk, overweight, or exhausted?
Of course, the negative things in your life, whether they're big or small, may
not go away today just because you take 5 minutes to focus on gratitude. But
try shifting your focus. Consider that your life right now, in this moment, has
sublime purpose.

Choose to recognize and name the pain or the funk. Instead of slamming
against it, imagine flowing with it like water moving around a rock. It doesn't
matter that the rock is there; the water finds its way, flowing with ease, grace,
direction, and purpose. Remember your intention today. Flow with your ups
and downs, and dance with your bumps and bruises.

How can you *choose* gratitude today, even though you may not feel it? Choose gratitude, and start to notice how your body feels. And remember, your challenges always bear gifts.

Today's Action Step: Make a Gratitude List

Make a list of 10 things in your life you're grateful for. Need some prompts? Try these: What's working? What's going really well? Who do you love? Who loves you? We're sure you can think of others.

Conscious Eating Meal Plan

Savoring your food and being mindful as you prepare a meal and eat it is a most important form of gratitude. In keeping with today's theme, try focusing on gratitude while you eat. This simple mental shift can be truly transformative. Happy cleansing!

Begin the day:

> Drink 1 quart warm lemon water.

Breakfast:

> Drink 1 quart your choice green smoothie. Try the Spicy Peach Smoothie.
>
> Or if it's cold outside or you're just hungry for a warm breakfast, try 1 or 2 cups Simple Breakfast Porridge.

Lunch:

> Feast on Colorful Collard Wraps with Zucchini Hummus, sliced avocado, and hemp seeds sprinkled on top.
>
> Want more protein? Add 4 to 8 ounces turkey breast, sliced, to the wrap.

Today's snack ideas:

> Nosh on 2 Protein-Packed Almond Butter Balls.
>
> Or sip some fresh green veggie juice (such as the Green Lemon Juice), or grab one from your local juice bar.
>
> You also could grab 2 to 4 ounces leftover Wild West Buffalo from a previous meal.

Dinner:

Salad Niçoise should do the trick.

If you want more protein, go with Baked Cod with Lemon and Olive Oil—and make extra for lunch this week!

End the day:

Sip at least 8 ounces warm lemon water.

Ingredient of the Day: Flaxseeds

Flaxseeds may not seem all that sexy, but boy do they pack a nutritional punch. They're a great source of fiber (the kind that makes your stool float), and they help with constipation. They also contain a good deal of omega-3 fatty acids and super-good-for-you phytochemicals called lignans. The omega-3s found in flaxseeds help lower the risk of heart disease and reduce inflammation. This wonder seed has also been shown to lower bad cholesterol (LDL) levels. In fact, a recent study showed that flaxseeds have comparable cholesterol-lowering benefits to pharmaceutical statin (cholesterol-lowering) drugs like Lipitor.

Big Business

A change in diet can naturally bring cholesterol levels to within a healthy range, but pharmaceutical statins—the class of drugs that inhibit cholesterol-producing enzymes—are at an all-time high. In fact, more than 20 million Americans take statins, and Lipitor was the worldwide top-selling drug in 2010.

You can buy flaxseeds whole or already ground. Whole flaxseeds have a longer shelf life, and you can quickly grind them when you need to use them. The preground flaxseeds go bad more quickly, so be sure you buy them in the refrigerator section or in a vacuum-sealed package. Use your coffee bean grinder to grind the seeds before you eat them because the whole seed is not easily absorbed. Store ground flaxseeds in a tightly sealed container in the refrigerator or freezer for up to 90 days so they don't go rancid.

Feeling Constipated?

To get things moving, add 2 tablespoons ground flaxseeds to your daily smoothie. Flaxseeds are a great source of soluble and insoluble fiber—the latter important to digestive health and cleansing—and support regular elimination. Flaxseeds are also rich in healthy omega-3 essential fatty acids, help the body metabolize fat stores, and help reduce inflammation. When buying flaxseeds, it's best to buy the whole flaxseed and grind it yourself, and bypass flaxseed meal.

Quick Tip: Water, Water, Water

The importance of drinking purified filtered water cannot be overstated. It's key to moving out the toxins and hydrating your body at a cellular level.

In our programs, we often hear, "Does tea count?" The answer is, "Nope!" Even with decaffeinated tea, your body has to filter the tea to get to the water. Your goal is to drink half your body weight in ounces of water each day, plus more if you exercise rigorously or live at a higher altitude.

Try drinking a glass of water at least 15 minutes before your next meal. Often, your hunger signal is actually just your body trying to tell you you're thirsty.

Constipated? Drink water! For many of you, the increase in fiber could possibly clog your pipes initially, so it's of supreme importance to hydrate to ease the flow.

Have you tried putting freshly squeezed lemon juice in your water yet? Besides being deliciously satisfying, it's exceptionally good for you. Lemon water helps flush fat out of your cells, alkalizes your body, and cleanses your liver. It's a natural digestive aid and an excellent source of vitamin C. Just take ½ lemon to 1 quart water. It's great to drink warm, but room temperature is fine, too. Try to avoid using ice if you can because it just creates another step for your body to warm the water so it can be absorbed and assimilated.

Need another way to drink it down? Sip warm water throughout the day *every 10 minutes.* Yep, that's right. Every 10 minutes, take a sip. Just carry around a to-go mug with you and sip warm water. This is the fastest way to hydrate your cells.

So what are you waiting for? Drink up!

In Your Journal

What are you grateful for? Make a list in your journal.

Day 5: Eat and Be Present

Surviving is important. Thriving is elegant.
—Maya Angelou

Whether you've been riding the highs or the lows of the process, today is a new day. Today is about hitting your stride and sailing into the weekend. Be sure to take the time to read the next chapter about the upcoming purification weekend. The gift of purification yields long-term benefits for your body, mind, and soul. So start to mentally prepare today. Get yourself to the grocery store so you have a fridge full of the green stuff ready and waiting for you.

Unsure about purification because of your weekend plans? Clear your schedule now. Give yourself space to rest and relax. You'll be so glad you did.

Today's conscious focus is perfect because by now you're probably green on the inside, free (hopefully) of those gnarly detox symptoms and sugar withdrawals and ready to take your consciousness to an entirely new level.

Conscious Focus: A Practice in Conscious Eating

For the past 4 days, you've been eating really good, wholesome foods, foods bursting with amazing flavors and natural tastes. But how much do you really *taste* your food? Think for a moment about where you eat most of your meals. Standing up? In the car? Watching TV? While you're working? At your computer?

Most of us feel there's just not enough time to keep up. As a result, we cram in eating while reading emails, watching TV, talking on the phone, texting, or driving. We eat standing up at the stove while cooking; we eat on our way from the stove to the table; we eat from the table back to the sink while cleaning up.

The net result is that we end up cheating ourselves of any possibility of pleasure or enjoyment from our food. What's worse is that when we eat mindlessly and quickly, we eat more, and we seriously mess with the digestion process, missing the part that happens in the mouth! Slowing down and really chewing your food allows the digestive juices that break down your food to be released.

Today's Action Step: Eat Without Distractions

Today's action is to eat just one meal without any distractions. That's right—*no* distractions. That means no TV, no radio, no computer, no texting, no smartphone, no conversation, no reading, no making to-do lists. Do nothing but eat, chew, taste, and be conscious of what happens next. After the first bite, what do you notice?

This can be a hard habit to break in the long run, but notice how you have to nearly sit on your hands to stop yourself from multitasking. Try putting down your fork (or smoothie) between bites. This simple pause is meditative and allows your body the chance to react on both a sensory and physiological level. If you're feeling really adventurous, try chewing each bite 25, 50, or even 100 times.

Have fun with this and take some time to journal about it. But not until you're done eating!

Conscious Eating Meal Plan

In preparation for purification, our meal suggestions are lighter and less filling. Feel free to follow our suggestions or follow your intuition.

Begin the day:

> Drink 1 quart warm lemon water.

Breakfast:

> Drink 1 quart your choice green smoothie. Try the Coco for Cilantro Smoothie.

Lunch:

> Enjoy a Golden Beet Salad.
> Or if you're feeling like a protein lover, try a simple chicken breast.
> Feeling like a grain lover? Enjoy the Golden Beet Salad on top of 1 cup cooked quinoa or buckwheat instead.

Today's snack ideas:

Snack on 1 cup cooked quinoa with juice of ½ lemon, sea salt, and pepper.

Or try some raw or lightly steamed veggies.

An apple or a pear also works.

Dinner:

Enjoy some Chilled Cucumber Dill Soup.

For a protein pick, how about some leftover cod from last night's dinner?

If you're still hungry, toss together a side salad with olive oil and lemon.

Watch the Clock

Be sure you have your last meal on Day 5 before 6 P.M. in preparation for your upcoming conscious purification.

End the day:

Sip at least 8 ounces warm lemon water.

Ingredient of the Day: Healthy Oils

Let's talk a minute about healthy oils. Hands down, these are the best oils to use:

- Borage oil
- Coconut oil
- Flaxseed oil
- Hemp seed oil
- Olive oil
- Sesame oil

Always buy *organic, cold-pressed unrefined oils* so you get oils that have not been heated or altered from their original state. Oils that have been heated have less nutritional value, are more processed, and usually have a less-robust flavor. For this reason, cold-pressed oils tend to be more expensive because they're technically a higher-quality oil.

Most of these oils are best used *after* you cook, so you can retain the healthy benefits they offer. That includes olive oil! (Surprising, we know.) But for example, if you're going to cook your veggies, it's best to steam or water-stir-fry them (see the Vegetable Medley Stir-Fry recipe for more info on this) and add the oil after. You'll use much less oil, you'll get the good benefits, and it's easier to clean the pan. Win-win-win.

When you need to cook with oils, the best types to use are sesame oil and coconut oil, which can withstand higher levels of heat.

Here are some of the brands of oils we love and recommend:

Nonheat oils:

> *Olive oil:* Biorganic, Spectrum, Bragg, David Wolfe Foods
>
> *Flaxseed oil:* Barlean's, Flora
>
> *Hemp seed oil:* Nutiva
>
> *Borage oil:* Spectrum, Barlean's

Oils for cooking:

> *Coconut oil:* Nutiva, Spectrum
>
> *Sesame oil:* Spectrum, Flora (be sure to find one that's not toasted)

Quick Tip: The Many Uses and Benefits of Coconut Oil

Not only is coconut oil one of the best oils to cook with, it also has some seriously profound healing properties. It has even been hailed as the healthiest oil on earth! Now that's a strong declaration! Oh, and did we mention coconut oil is the world's only natural low-calorie fat? Yeah, coconut oil rocks.

It's not just for cooking, either. Toss out your fancy, expensive skin-care products, and use coconut oil just like you would any moisturizer. Your skin will thank you. And since your skin is your largest organ, you'll be absorbing it and getting many of the same healing benefits you'd get if you ate it. Speaking of benefits, according to Dr. Joseph Mercola at the Natural Health Center, research has shown coconut oil to …

- Improve heart health.
- Boost the thyroid.
- Support healthy metabolism.

- Strengthen the immune system.
- Reduce inflammation.
- Give you quick and immediate energy.
- Promote weight loss when needed.
- Promote stable blood sugar.
- Support natural pH of the skin.
- Soften and protect the skin.
- Promote skin elasticity.
- Help relieve dryness and itching.
- Provide protection from UV rays.

That's quite an accomplishment for a humble oil!

In Your Journal

How do you usually eat? Hurried? Do you enjoy your food? Do you see it as a chore or something else on your list of to-do's? Write about this.

Intermezzo: Purification Weekend Guidelines

You're on your own.
And you know what you know.
And YOU are the one who'll decide where to go.

—Dr. Seuss

Welcome to the first conscious purification weekend! Your mission, should you choose to accept it, is to consume only vegetables and fruits, with no more than 2 tablespoons of oil, for the next 2 days. The key to your success, enjoyment, and fulfillment here is *rest!*

Purification Guidelines

Here are the basic guidelines for your first purification weekend. In a nutshell, your goal is to eat only vegetables and fruits, using a small amount of oil for added flavor (and healthy fat).

- Eat as many vegetables and fruits as you desire.
- Veggies can be raw or lightly steamed.
- Try to keep your vegetable-to-fruit ratio at 3:1.
- Drink unlimited freshly squeezed vegetable and fruit juices or smoothies.
- Limit yourself to 2 tablespoons of a healthy oil of your choice per day.
- Keep it simple.

Beginning and Ending Your Purification

If you started the Conscious Cleanse on a Monday, purification will fall on Saturday and Sunday. If your weekends are jam-packed and it makes more sense for you to do it on Sunday and Monday, that's fine. The key is to find 2 days, back to back, around your halfway point, when you can rest, relax, and reflect.

Purification technically begins after your last meal on Day 5. Try to finish eating by 6 P.M. that evening.

Purification ends on the evening of Day 7. With dinner, add 2 to 4 ounces animal or vegetable protein and 1 or 2 tablespoons oil—that's all—to your regular purification meal. This ends your purification gently and ensures you don't wake up ready to eat the entire contents of your refrigerator. This evening meal transitions you back to conscious eating for another 5 days.

Caring for Yourself During Purification

Think of purification as a mini-wellness retreat, and take care of yourself the way you would if you were at a five-star spa resort.

One of the things you should do on this purification weekend is to prepare and enjoy Bieler's Broth. This healing soup was created by Dr. Henry Bieler, a clinical nutritionist and author of the book *Food Is Your Best Medicine*. The soup is bright green and very bland by nature, and as you may have guessed, therein lies its healing properties. The soup is rich in minerals and is very alkalizing. You may be tempted to spice it up with sea salt or other spices, but keeping it bland actually helps you recalibrate your taste buds. It's nourishing, restorative, comforting, and fulfilling. Enjoy it frequently throughout your purification. (We give you the recipe in Part 4.)

Another recipe to try during your purification is our Spicy Lemon Elixir. Drink it in the morning and up to five times throughout the day. This drink is an offshoot of the Master Cleanse drink from the 1940s, but without the sugar. It's refreshing and satisfying to the taste buds, and the cayenne kick helps stimulate your digestive fire.

Rest is another important component of the purification. It's a must for detoxification. Plan ahead and cancel all unnecessary activities. Hire a babysitter, sleep late, take naps, read books, and go to bed early. If you follow this simple advice, your hunger and discomfort will be greatly reduced. And use the downtime to tap into your body's inherent healing wisdom!

Another thing to remember is that if you feel hungry, you should eat. Vegetables and fruits digest very quickly, so you may find yourself eating every couple hours or eating more than three square meals. That's okay. Eat when you're hungry.

It's important to stay hydrated, too. Drink lots of water and other liquids like herbal tea infusions and veggie juices. How do you know if you're drinking enough? Try to have 10 clear pees throughout the day.

If you experience symptoms such as headache, fatigue, mood swings, nervousness, or nausea ... *get excited!* These symptoms are the result of the toxic substances being pulled from your cells and tissues into your bloodstream for elimination. This means your purification is working! The best thing to do if you experience these feelings is rest and drink lots of liquids. We give you more tips on how to manage detox symptoms on Day 6.

Partial Purification and Special Circumstances

Going along with our theme that this is not an all-or-nothing proposition, we want to acknowledge that there are always special circumstances when the full-blown purification may not be right for you at this time. If you're training for a marathon, nursing an infant, not wanting to lose weight, have an event you can't cancel, or another special circumstance, consider customizing your purification in a way that rests your digestive system *and* works for your current situation.

A partial purification could look a number of different ways. Find the way that works best for you. Here are some examples:

- Eat just veggies and fruits for breakfast and lunch, or two thirds of the day. At dinner, introduce a small amount of protein (2 to 4 ounces only), ½ cup grains, a handful of nuts, or ½ an avocado.

- Eat only fruits and vegetables, but supplement more with the slower-digesting foods like avocados or coconut oil. Both are great additions to a green smoothie.

Whatever you do, do your best and listen to your body. Commit *and* be flexible, loving, and smart.

The idea of purification may sound terrifying to you. We understand, because we've been there. Know that a partial purification is a viable option, but also proceed with courage. You can do this. And you might be surprised that it's not as challenging in reality as it might seem in your head.

Note some people should not do this purification, not even the partial version. If you have an eating disorder, you're pregnant, or your current health is too weak, purification is not for you. If you're currently under a physician's care, be sure you consult your doctor before starting purification.

Day 6:
Purification Weekend 1

Our deepest fear is not that we are inadequate.
Our deepest fear is that we are powerful beyond
measure.

—Marianne Williamson

Are you ready to be a lean, green, guzzling machine? To infuse your body
with fresh vegetables, fruits, and live enzymes? Are you ready to feel refreshed
and renewed? The journey of purification starts now. It takes tremendous
courage to show up here, so just commit to doing your personal best, and
remember your best is good enough!

Today we're going to talk about feelings. Yeah, yeah, yeah, we know—not
everyone's favorite topic. Most of us have pretty much become masters of
"taking the emotion out of it." But let's face it: giving yourself a rest from your
usual food routine is going to bring up some stuff. Or at least, that's the hope.

So decide right now that you're going to allow yourself to feel whatever comes
up for you today. Notice if you start to feel more emotionally vulnerable.
Pay very close attention to the emotions that come up during this time, be it
sadness, anger, frustration, annoyance, silliness, or orneriness. Take a deep
breath, and instead of indulging your instincts to run or push down these big
emotions with food, sit someplace quiet and feel into them.

We know this is easier said than done. But we also know you can do it. May
the force be with you this weekend.

Conscious Focus: Creating Your Own Wellness Retreat

Part of making the most of your purification weekend is creating a space for yourself to have a mini-retreat—or a *stay-cation*, as we like to say. Pampering yourself this weekend will yield long-term health benefits for your body, mind, and spirit. Enjoy some R&R, lie on the couch, watch a good movie, journal, laugh, take slow walks, or whatever pleases you. And above all, *rest, rest, rest!*

What do you do in your life currently to pamper yourself that doesn't involve food? Most of us eat to comfort ourselves, to reward ourselves, or to soothe ourselves. This weekend, we want you to find other ways to care for yourself. If you haven't done this before, it may feel a bit indulgent or uncomfortable. You're probably used to giving lots to others, allowing yourself to fall by the wayside.

This weekend, imagine yourself as a small child. How would you care for a little you? How would you talk to yourself? What would you do for this small child? Do that for yourself this weekend.

Today's Action Step: Relax and Enjoy "Doing" Nothing

One of our favorite ways to feel pampered is to create a space that feels relaxing. The best way to do this is by taking a hot bath! Prepare a hot bath today by using 1 cup of Epsom salts and a few drops of lavender essential oil. Dim the lights, put on some relaxing music, light a few candles, soak, and relax. Or sit outside in the fresh air. Feel the sun on your skin. Put your toes in the grass, and feel the ground.

Take moments throughout the day to really stop and feel this day, this hour, this minute, and this moment. Allow this time to deeply nourish and revitalize you.

Conscious Purification Meal Plan

The theme for eating during purification is *keep it simple*. Forget the fancy recipes, and eat real, simple, fresh, wholesome, life-giving food.

Begin the day:

Drink 1 quart warm lemon water.

Breakfast:

Drink 1 quart your choice green smoothie plus ½ tablespoon your favorite oil. For example, make a Dandy Dandelion Smoothie and add ½ tablespoon coconut oil.

Watch Your Oil

Choose a smoothie without seeds, nut milks, or avocado. If the smoothie recipe calls for more than 2 tablespoons oil, remember this is your oil for the entire day. We recommend you spread out your oil intake. Cut the recipe's suggested amount to ½ to 1 tablespoon oil instead.

Lunch:

Make a large salad with 1 tablespoon your favorite oil in a dressing. Need a suggestion? The Rainbow Salad with Citrus Squeeze Dressing is great. Again, watch your oil intake. Remember, you're only eating 2 tablespoons for the day in total.

Today's snack ideas:

Go for a Green Mango Smoothie.

Sliced veggies or a piece of fruit also make a great snack.

Or drink Bieler's Broth or our Spicy Lemon Elixir.

Dinner:

Make a huge bowl of lightly steamed veggies with ½ tablespoon oil.

Or make a huge plate of steamed kale topped with Vegetable Medley Stir-Fry. Flavor with ½ tablespoon olive oil.

End the day:

Sip at least 8 ounces warm lemon water.

Ingredient of the Day: Sprouts

By now, you know we are suckers for anything that packs a nutrient punch, so it only makes sense that we take a moment to talk about sprouts. Sprouting is a process by which you soak a seed, grain, or bean in water over a period of time, converting it into a tasty, easily digested food. The most readily available sprouts found at your local grocery store are alfalfa, broccoli, clover, mung bean, radish, and sunflower sprouts. It's good to use a variety of sprouts on salads, in wraps, and even in green smoothies.

Sprouts are bursting with enzymes, minerals, phytonutrients, protein, and vitamins, especially C. They're known as a "high-energy food" because the body is able to quickly convert them into usable energy.

Growing your own sprouts is an easy and inexpensive way to have fresh, living food growing right on your countertop (in a jar, that is) all year long. All you need is a glass jar, a drying rack, some fresh seeds, and pure filtered water.

Feeling Hungry?

What does hunger feel like in your body? Most of us hardly ever feel true hunger anymore. We eat according to the clock, we eat because we're angry or sad, or we eat because the kids are eating. Getting in touch with your hunger can be a very powerful experience. Now, this isn't about depriving or starving yourself from a place of punishment or as a means of battling your willpower. This is about tuning in to your body and listening to what it needs at a deeper level.

During purification, you eat quick-digesting, light, high-vibration foods. The result is that you feel lighter, more open, and more energized. Notice what it feels like to not be stuffed after every meal. Notice how you feel physically, and watch what surfaces emotionally.

Feeling raw and open is a good thing. If you feel like crying for no reason, or find yourself getting irritated by something insignificant, stay with what's surfacing—what now has space to surface. Allow it all to bubble up so you can release it, and let it go. Often the extra weight we carry around is a protective layer. When we deal with old hurt or trauma, the pounds begin to melt away.

When Jo did purification for the first time, she remembers how unexpected the process was for her. It was 4 p.m. on Saturday, the first day of purification, and all she could think about was a chicken breast. How weird! A chicken breast isn't typically something she'd crave, let alone obsess about. So she decided to lie on the couch, rest, relax, and take care of herself.

At that moment, her boyfriend walked into the room, so she whined to him about how all she wanted was a chicken breast. She was so flustered. He responded by telling her she should just go eat a chicken breast. It was in that very moment that she had her mini-epiphany. Bursting into tears, she exclaimed, "But it's not about the chicken breast!"

That her boyfriend left the room shaking his head in bewilderment is beside the point. The point is: notice what your chicken breast is this weekend. Ask yourself if it's really about the food. What are you really hungry for? What do you really need in that moment?

Quick Tip: Dealing with Detox

Although detox doesn't always feel great, let yourself rejoice at some level because it means you're getting the toxins out! It may not be easy, but it's an achievement in and of itself to find gratitude in a moment of discomfort.

Here are some signs and symptoms you might be detoxing:

- Acne or small breakouts
- Diarrhea
- Fatigue
- Gas
- Headaches
- Irritability
- Low energy
- Mood swings
- Skin rashes

And here are some tips for easing the pain or discomfort of detox:

- Rest.
- Do little to no physical activity except for a leisurely stroll in the sunshine.
- Drink *a lot* of water.
- Take a hot Epsom salt bath. Be sure to dunk your head, especially if you have a headache.
- Do a dry brush scrub. Use a dry washcloth, and work from your feet up, moving toward your heart.
- Jump up and down, use a trampoline, or rebound in place.
- Get a massage.
- Rest, rest, rest!

In Your Journal

What's underneath your hunger? What are you really feeling? What do you really need from yourself today?

Day 7: Cleansing from the Outside In

The state of your life is nothing more than a reflection of your state of mind.

—Dr. Wayne W. Dyer

What's so amazing about cleansing yourself on the inside is the natural spill-over effect. You know what we mean—the spontaneous desire to finally wash your car, clean out the junk drawer, reorganize your closet, or donate that growing pile of clothes you don't wear anymore.

As you're taking on purification and disconnecting a bit from food and all the baggage that comes with it, the opportunity to reconnect with a deeper place in yourself, your environment, and the people around you arises. Notice how the sky looks bluer and how you can listen with more openness to your loved ones.

We think it's pretty darn amazing to recalibrate your taste buds, but hitting the reboot button on your entire life and all your relationships ... now *that's* out of this world! That's the power of purification.

Conscious Focus: Detox Your Environment

Ever heard the saying, "How a person manages their stuff is the same way they manage their emotions"? Take a look around at your living space today. Look really closely. Are mounds of dust piling up in the corners of the hall-way? Could your tub use a good scrubbing? Does your refrigerator or do your kitchen cabinets need cleaning and organizing? Look around your office or workspace. Is your keyboard dirty? Your file cabinet messy? How's the garage or the basement? How about your inbox? What's your stuff telling you?

Most of us have a "dirty little secret" somewhere in our homes. We like to call it the "catch-all." What are you tossing into the catch-all to deal with another time? Do you realize the undercurrent of annoyance it causes? Can you feel how it weighs you down?

Believe it or not, the way you manage your stuff is the same way you likely manage your not-so-pleasant emotions. You toss them aside, stuff them with food, and avoid them at all costs.

We love the saying "How you do anything is how you do everything." Think about that. When you fold your towels, do you then stuff them into the too-small bathroom cabinet instead of taking the time to reorganize it so they all fit nicely? What else are you stuffing in your life? What else are you hanging on to that you need to deal with?

As you move deeper into cleansing yourself from the inside out, naturally you'll feel the urge to take better care of everything else in your life. And the feeling of finally wrapping up some unfinished business or of giving your closet a good purge will leave you feeling lighter and more energized—purified from the outside in!

Today's Action Step: Clean Up Your Space

Take a look around your living and working space today. Ask yourself, *What is my stuff trying to tell me?* Take some small steps toward detoxing your external environment. If you're overwhelmed, just choose one place to start. Remember, nothing happens all at once. One step today, one step tomorrow. Just like the cleanse.

When our stuff is clean and organized, our thoughts are clear and focused. And when our thoughts are clear and focused, our emotions are real and authentic. The net result is a better, more balanced, fulfilling life. Hooray!

Conscious Wellness Evaluation Redux

Remember to revisit your Conscious Wellness Evaluation today. Cover up Day 1's answers, and rate yourself without comparing how you feel today with the beginning of the week. Just look at the evaluation with fresh eyes.

Conscious Purification Sample Meal Plan

Remember to focus on simplicity. Eat slowly and enjoy your food in its natural state—it's amazing how good it tastes unaltered, without anything covering it up. You'll note that we begin to ease you out of the purification weekend during the dinner meal, where we'll add a small amount of protein to avoid shocking your system tomorrow.

Begin the day:

> Drink 1 quart warm lemon water.

Breakfast:

> Drink 1 quart your choice green smoothie with 1 tablespoon oil.
> Maybe make the Apple Salad Smoothie with 1 tablespoon flaxseed oil.

Remember, Watch Your Oil

As mentioned in the previous chapter, remember to choose a smoothie without seeds, nut milks, or avocado on purification days. If the smoothie recipe calls for more than 2 tablespoons oil, remember this is your oil for the entire day. Cut the recipe's suggested amount to ½ to 1 tablespoon oil if need be.

Lunch:

> Eat a huge salad. The Super Big Easy Salad with 1½ tablespoons Italian Herb Dressing should do the trick. (Modify the dressing by taking out the mustard and honey to make it "purification" friendly, and add water instead.)

Today's snack ideas:

> Drink 1 quart Fasting Tea.
> Or nibble on some Fruit Salad Supreme.
> Or opt for a bowl of lightly steamed broccoli and cauliflower with a lemon squeeze.

Dinner:

> To ease out of your purification, add in 2 to 4 ounces protein (animal or vegetable) with an extra 1 or 2 tablespoons oil. For example, try Bieler's Broth drizzled with 1 or 2 tablespoons olive oil and 2 to 4 ounces baked

wild salmon or some sunflower seeds. (Sprinkle the sunflower seeds on top of Bieler's Broth.)

End the day:

Sip at least 8 ounces warm lemon water.

Ingredient of the Day: Nettle Leaf

Also known as stinging nettle or the "wonder weed," the nettle plant can be found growing all over the world. And while it's true, as the name suggests, that you want to be mindful when dealing with the actual plant, the nettle leaf is a powerful herb to incorporate into your diet today.

Herbalists (practitioners who use herbs medicinally) have used nettles in teas, infusions, and tinctures to strengthen and clean the blood, brighten the whites of the eyes, give the skin a healthy glow, and make hair shinier. Some even swear by nettles' ability to stimulate the growth of hair in balding men!

The list of healing benefits of this little green herb goes on:

- Assists the body in detoxing chemicals, especially heavy metals
- Helps with PMS symptoms and water retention
- Is anti-inflammatory and helps reduce pain associated with bursitis, rheumatoid arthritis, and gout
- Helps with hay fever and allergies because of its natural antihistamines
- Helps stimulate mother's milk production and restores energy after childbirth
- Is high in iron, calcium, magnesium, beta-carotene, boron, and silicon and is a good source of protein and the vitamins A, C, D, and B complex
- Boosts testosterone, increasing men's vitality

Experimenting with Nettles

If you're currently taking any medication, be sure to consult with your doctor before taking nettles because they can interact negatively. Check out Part 4 for a variety of herbal infusion recipes containing nettles. This is a great elixir to enjoy anytime, especially during purification.

Detoxing Your Household Cleaners

Want to greatly reduce your body's toxic load? Give your household cleaners an overhaul. Did you know that the average U.S. home contains between 3 and 25 gallons of toxic materials? Most of these are common, everyday household cleaning supplies.

The scary thing is, no laws keep you safe from such hazardous materials. Manufacturers are not required to list ingredients on their labels. As a consumer, you need to advocate for your own nontoxic environment. Read the labels of your usual household cleaners, and make the switch today to toxin-free cleaners.

Here are some of the culprits to avoid:

Ammonia   Fatal when ingested.

Butyl cellosolve   Damages bone marrow, the nervous system, kidneys, and the liver. Found in all-purpose, window, and other types of cleaners.

Chlorinated phenols   Toxic to respiratory and circulatory systems. Found in toilet bowl cleaners.

Diethylene glycol   Suppresses the nervous system. Found in window cleaners.

Formaldehyde   Respiratory irritant and suspected carcinogen. Found in spray and wick deodorizers.

Nonylphenol ethoxylate   Known as surfactants, or chemicals that grab dirt, nonylphenol ethoxylate is found in laundry detergents and all-purpose cleaners. It lingers around the environment, gets into the water supply, and is toxic to the ecosystem. It's banned in Europe.

Perchloroethylene   Damaging to the liver and kidneys. Found in spot removers.

Petroleum solvent   Destroys mucous membranes. Found in floor cleaners.

Phenols   Toxic to respiratory and circulatory systems. Found in disinfectants.

This list is by no means complete, so look at all your cleaning supplies. If the label contains the words *warning, danger, caution,* or *poison,* give it the old heave-ho! Products that contain bleach, phosphates, petroleum, lye, and chlorine are also no good!

The good news—yes, we do have some!—is that there are amazing alternatives out there. Some of our favorite nontoxic cleaners come from Seventh Generation, Earth Friendly Products, and Dr. Bronner's. An even better option is to make your own! It's easy and more cost effective.

Quick Tip: Making Nontoxic Household Cleaners

If you're feeling a bit overwhelmed and ready to toss all the toxic cleansers in your house, you're going to need replacements. Making your own is simple and time-tested. It's what Grandma used to clean with!

Furniture Polish
Yield: about 1 cup

2 tsp. olive or jojoba oil

1 cup fresh lemon juice

In a glass jar with a tight-fitting lid, combine olive oil and lemon juice. Dip a cloth rag into the polish, and wipe your wood surfaces.

All-Purpose Cleaner/Wood Floor Cleaner
Yield: about 2 cups

1 cup white vinegar

1 cup water

In a spray bottle, combine white vinegar and water. Use throughout the house just like you would an all-purpose cleaner on all types of surfaces. Don't worry—the vinegar smell will go away.

Tub and Tile Cleaner
Yield: about 3 cups

$1^2/_3$ cups baking soda

$1/_2$ cup vegetable oil–based liquid soap

$1/_2$ cup water

2 TB. white vinegar

In a jar or spray bottle, combine baking soda, liquid soap, water, and white vinegar. Shake well before using. Apply with a cloth or sponge, and rinse well.

Mold and Mildew Remover _____
Yield: about 2 cups

2 tsp. tea tree oil
2 cups water

In a spray bottle, combine tea tree oil and water. Use on moldy shower curtains, musty rugs, or moldy furniture. This works great on yoga mats, too!

In Your Journal

What in your life could use some clutter-busting? What can you get rid of? What needs to be organized or cleaned out?

Day 8:
Refresh and Renew

Our greatest glory is not in never falling but in rising
every time we fall.

—Confucius

Welcome to Week 2! How are you feeling today? Did you tackle purification? You've officially crossed the halfway point! Congratulations! Today is a great day to really step back and take note of any changes you're experiencing. During Day 7, you revisited the wellness survey from the beginning of the book and compared how you feel now versus when you started. Let's think about that some more.

It's so interesting to us how often our participants forget just how crummy they may have felt a short week ago. So take note of your experience now to fully own it. Really think about all the power that comes from the simple act of eating real food.

Today is about hitting the refresh button. The halfway point offers a nice symmetry to begin thinking about the larger vision. As you know, we love the saying, "The way you do *anything* is the way you do *everything*." We believe strongly that the way you eat is a reflection of the way you live your life. So this week, we'll begin to dive deeper into one of our favorite topics: *soul food*. Believe it or not, what's on your plate, green and glorious as it may be, is only part of the picture.

Conscious Focus: Soul Food

Say it once again with us: "Food is never just about food." But have you ever really stopped to think what else it *is* about? Why does food lend itself so well to being an emotional response? How is it that food can be both our go-to reward for ourselves and our punishment? There must be something else to it, something profound, something that goes beyond the food on our plates that has the power to make us feel good or bad.

Today we want to explore how you're feeding your soul. What things bring you joy, fulfillment, peace, and a sense of purpose, and how can you feed these things in the same way you're working to feed the physical systems of your body? This is the essence of soul food. Malnourishment of your soul all too often bleeds into the use and abuse of real food. This is a natural way of masking the pain associated with gaps we sometimes feel in other areas of our lives.

There are four main categories of soul food:

- Physical activity
- Fulfilling work
- Relationships
- Spirituality

Let's take a closer look at each of these.

Your body thrives on movement—doing yoga, going for a walk, playing catch or kicking a ball with a child, riding a bike, etc. It doesn't have to feel like "exercise." And it shouldn't feel like a chore to be endured, but rather a respite from the day—something you look forward to. It doesn't matter what it is, just find something (or multiple somethings!) you love to do and integrate it into your day, every day.

Having a purpose-driven life, a career you love, or simply finding a way to love the work you're currently doing all constitute fulfilling work. Being willing to truly shift your perspective or recognizing when it's time to let go of something you're used to is scary stuff, but it's all part of this thing called life.

When we talk about relationships, we don't just mean romantic ones. Friends, family, parents, children, co-workers, teachers, neighbors—how you deal with others is how you deal with yourself. Healthy relationships support you at your core and make you feel like you're not alone. Healing an unresolved relationship is far more beneficial to your overall well-being than any amount of spinach you can eat.

Finally, having a connection to a power outside yourself is fundamental to the experience of gratitude. Being grateful for your life and the things in it can help put a lot of things in perspective. Your stress decreases, and you have a sense of ease. It doesn't matter what you call it—God, nature, life force, energy, breath—it's all good. Learning to quiet your mind, to find peace and reverence in the everyday, is key to living a balanced and fulfilling life.

Food for the Soul

Just as food is needed for the body, love is needed for the soul.

—Osho

Today's Action Step: Feed Your Soul

What feeds your soul? Rate yourself in the four categories of soul food we described earlier—physical activity, fulfilling work, relationships, and spirituality—on a scale of 1 to 10 with 1 being dissatisfied and 10 being your version of perfection.

Now, do one thing in the area where you gave yourself the lowest number. Big or small, drastic or subtle—take positive action today.

Conscious Eating Meal Plan

As you transition into Week 2, we suggest even more of a plant-based diet, with fewer grains and fewer animal protein options. Give it a try, and if you feel like you need to supplement with a grain or an animal protein, by all means, eat! Consider having less of these foods, though (½ cup grains versus 1 cup, for example), and more of the plant-based options.

Begin the day:

Drink 1 quart warm lemon water.

Breakfast:

Drink 1 quart your choice green smoothie. We suggest the Creamy Cherry Smoothie.

Lunch:

A lunch of Simple Basil Pesto Zucchini Pasta with Chopped Italian Salad sounds perfect.

Today's snack ideas:

> Nibble on 3 or 4 Joy Balls.
>
> Or enjoy a Chickpea Hummus wrap.
>
> Or try Tropical Mango Salsa with Carrot Chips.

Dinner:

> What's for dinner? How about Buckwheat Arame with Citrus Burst Broccoli?
>
> If you're craving protein, instead of the Buckwheat Arame, try your broccoli with Broiled Lamb Chops.

End the day:

> Sip at least 8 ounces warm lemon water.

Ingredient of the Day: Chia Seeds

The chia seed, which has been around so long even the Aztecs used it as their main energy source, comes from a small flowering plant in the mint family.

These tiny little seeds are similar to flaxseeds but with some subtle differences. They contain healthy fats, and they're packed with protein, antioxidants, soluble fiber, and tons of healthy vitamins and minerals often lacking in normal diets. Chia seeds can help restore energy levels and decrease inflammation because of their omega-3 fatty acids.

Similar to cornstarch, chia seeds can be used as a thickening agent and as a substitute for whole grains in your diet. Whole grains help stabilize your blood sugar levels, as opposed to the spikes and falls that result from consuming sugar and refined carbohydrates.

Chia seeds also help with:

- Anti-aging
- Improved moods
- Good cholesterol
- Joint and pain relief
- Decreased food cravings

Chia seeds come in either black or white varieties, and there's no difference in taste or nutritional value between the two. Chia seeds can be used in smoothies; sprinkled on salads; or ground and added to flaxseed crackers, homemade applesauce, or dessert puddings (see the Better-Than-Yogurt Chia Pudding recipe). And kids love chia seeds!

Soak for Success

We recommend soaking your chia seeds for at least 15 minutes before adding them to your smoothie or favorite recipe. In a small glass jar, cover ¼ cup (or desired amount) chia seeds with water to cover. The chia seeds will absorb the water to make a gel-like consistency. This will keep in the fridge for a few days.

Quick Tip: Maximizing Weight Loss

Although weight loss is secondary to the benefits of feeling better in the Conscious Cleanse, we recognize that it's often a highly desired secondary benefit! So here are a few more tips to help your body "release" the weight:

Be sure you're getting enough sleep. According to Michael Breus, PhD, author of *The Sleep Doctor's Diet*, losing just 1 hour of sleep for 3 consecutive days can promote a surge in the hormone ghrelin, which actually stimulates appetite. When you get deep sleep, you also produce more of the fat-burning human growth hormone (HGH).

Look at your stress levels. When you feel high levels of stress, you release a hormone called cortisol. Cortisol can actually cue your body to want high-carbohydrate foods. If you can't immediately control your stress levels, it's important to be aware that these cravings can be brought on by stress. More importantly, it's crucial to learn techniques to take the stress out of your life: deep breathing, yoga, meditation, exercise, walking in nature, and unplugging from your electronics are all great ways to start.

Get moving! If you haven't started to make exercise part of your daily routine, begin to think about how you can move more. Take the stairs. Ask a friend to go for a walk instead of getting a drink (which you aren't having anyway!). Try a new exercise class, or take a dance class. It doesn't have to be hard or overwhelming. And just like with diet, small changes add up in major ways.

Stop weighing yourself! Throw out your scale, or at least hide it for the next week. We have had past participants who were getting on the scale daily and measured their success by pounds lost. This unhealthy tendency is an unnecessary obsession that can do little but stress you out. Remember what stress does to weight loss? Don't worry: you *will* "release" weight! Focus on the benefits you're seeing already after just 1 week. Equally profound surprises await you in Week 2 and beyond!

Get Off the Roller Coaster

If you've been on the roller-coaster ride of a chronic dieter, you may need a bit longer for results to kick in due to the effects of that roller coaster on your metabolism. Be patient. Keep going. Do what feels good, and the weight loss will follow—guaranteed!

Consider other food sensitivities. Although we've eliminated the heavy-hitting allergens, it's still possible that you're eating foods that you're sensitive to. We've had participants who noticed that they couldn't tolerate avocados, coconuts, grains, lentils, mangos, and other nuts. Be curious. Notice any compulsions for certain foods. Consider taking those out for a few days to see if you feel better or "release weight." Remember foods that you are sensitive to can cause inflammation and water retention, even if it is a "healthy food."

Eat mindfully. This week you learned how to slow down and eat to actually taste your food. Continue to make it a practice every day to eat slowly, to notice when you're full. A full belly isn't the goal. If you eat nuts for a snack, don't go for the whole bag. You can overdo a good thing! Bottom line: eat when you're hungry and stop when you're full. This will result in life-long weight management. Seems simple enough, right?

Finally, eat an early dinner. Many of us eat late-night meals or snacks, whether you work late, feel hungry, or just can't shake the habit. Studies have shown that eating after 8 P.M. can cause weight gain and an increase in your body mass index. To lose weight, try eating before 8 P.M.

In Your Journal

What feeds your soul? What area of your soul food needs some healing or attention? What is one action you can take today to give that area of your life some extra attention?

Day 9: Conscious Moxie

> You yourself, as much as anybody in the entire universe, deserve your love and affection.
>
> —Buddha

Going along with this week's theme of ways to create whole-body health, our focus today is on beauty and self-care. We love this point in our program, because as you cleanse from the inside out, it's only natural that it begins to show up on the outside. This is typically when participants report that their friends and family start to notice they have a certain glow about them. It's true that eating more vegetables and fruits actually does directly affect your skin tone, but the glow, as you've probably noticed, also comes from a deeper place.

When you feel good in your skin and in your body, it's natural to want to reflect that. You'll feel the urge to shower, shave, wash, *and* maybe even— *gasp!—style your hair*. So go ahead! Feel free to put on sexy clothes, even if you're working from home or running errands. Feel your moxie. Explore your mojo. When you're feeling groovy, the call to spiff up is simply an outpouring of the good vibrations you have on the inside.

Conscious Focus: Self-Care and Pampering

In the hurried pace of day-to-day life, it can be so easy to put ourselves last. I mean really, who has time to eat well, exercise, *and* pamper themselves? Seriously! Even small luxuries—a manicure, taking time to read a book—can seem extravagant. And it's a truly lucky day if we don't feel the need to be on our smartphones multitasking our ways through the hours.

Well, today we're going to make up for some lost time. There are many, many ways you can pamper yourself. Practicing good self-care may be as simple as showering and putting on some clothes that make you feel good. It's amazing what this simple act can do to lift your spirits. Other things to consider include getting a massage, taking a bubble bath (you already know how much we love these!), giving yourself a clay mask facial, giving your hair a natural oil treatment (coconut oil with some essential oils works great), or try dry brushing from head to toe to scrape off some dead skin.

This goes for the men, too! Get dressed, try a professional shave, sit in the sauna, or get a rubdown. Don't be afraid to treat yourself right!

Choosing Skin-Care Products

Joshua Scott Onysko, founder and CEO of Pangea Organics, says: "The skin is the largest organ of the human body. It not only protects us from infections and bacteria, it often reflects the overall health of our being. For me, caring for the skin has always been a ritual, much like sitting down to a fine meal. Balancing the skin is as much about mental and internal health as the quality and integrity of the products we put on it. An easy rule of thumb when deciding what skin-care products to use is to look at the ingredients, and if you cannot pronounce the ingredient names and/or would not eat them, then they are probably not good for you."

Today's Action Step: Date Night

Make a date with yourself tonight, and do something that pampers *you*. We know you have many to-dos and lots of things that normally come ahead of "you" on the priority list, but for today, plan on putting yourself first!

Conscious Eating Meal Plan

In Week 2, we continue to ask you (and your taste buds) to be a bit more adventurous. The smoothies are getting greener and the meal plan even cleaner, with less cooked food and more raw, living food options. Remember to be open and flexible. Consider giving the meal plan a try, but if it's not suiting your needs, follow your intuition, and adjust accordingly.

Begin the day:

> Drink 1 quart warm lemon water.

Breakfast:

> Drink 1 quart your choice green smoothie. Need an idea? Try the Pink 'n' Green Smoothie.

Lunch:

Sample the Caesar Salad or the Red Ruby Trout Salad.

Today's snack ideas:

Beet Hummus with veggie of choice would work.

Or maybe Raw Trail Mix is more your speed today.

A sliced avocado topped with dulse flakes would also hit the spot.

Dinner:

Make a Kale Seaweed Salad, and serve it over 1 or 2 cups brown rice.

End the day:

Sip at least 8 ounces warm lemon water.

Ingredient of the Day: Sea Vegetables

The thought of sea vegetables probably conjures up an image of the gloppy green stuff we try to avoid when walking on the beach or swimming in the ocean. But seaweeds, a.k.a. sea vegetables, are ocean plants that have been harvested for centuries and used in the daily diet of many coastal cultures around the world.

We consider sea vegetables superfoods—and integral to vibrant health because of their unparalleled array of minerals, phytonutrients, and vitamins. They are, in fact, among the most nutrient-dense foods on the planet!

While the introduction of sea vegetables may seem foreign or daunting at first, fret not. We give you some tasty recipes in Part 4 that will help you make friends with this superfood.

Success with Sea Vegetables

Sea vegetables need to be soaked in water for about 15 to 20 minutes before using. You can also use dulse flakes as a yummy addition to soups or salads. These days, sea vegetables are typically available at most grocery stores and health food stores. For a greater selection, you might want to try a local Asian market.

Here are some different types of sea vegetables generally available:

- Arame
- Dulse
- Hijiki
- Kelp
- Kombu
- Nori
- Wakame

Incorporating sea vegetables into your diet has been proven to have significant health benefits. Sea vegetables ...

- Are anti-inflammatory.
- Are a good source of minerals, especially iodine and iron.
- Help alkalize the blood.
- Improve digestion.
- Reduce blood cholesterol.
- Reduce cravings.
- Stabilize blood sugar.
- Strengthen hair and nails.
- Are one of the richest plant sources of calcium.
- Improve liver function.
- Help maintain a healthy, functioning thyroid.
- Lower blood pressure.

Iodine Deficiency

Iodine deficiency is a worldwide concern. In the United States, where we've been taught all salt is bad, we've gotten into a bit of a salt predicament. Salt is essential to life, but you must use the right kind. Some sea salts are highly refined, and many contain little or no iodine, which can create deficiencies. Some signs of iodine deficiency include chronic fatigue, apathy, dry skin, cold intolerance, weight gain, and thyroid (goiter) enlargement. To avoid deficiency, add sea vegetables to your diet and switch to high-quality salt, like Himalayan or Celtic sea salt.

Quick Tip: What's in Your Beauty Products?

Forgive us for a moment while we get on our soapbox about this topic. Cosmetics include everything from makeup (blush, lipstick, foundation, powder, mascara, eye liner, etc.) to skin-care lotions and face creams, to hair dyes, nail polish, and perfumes. It also includes such everyday products as deodorants, shampoos, bubble bath, soap, hair spray, hair gels, and hand sanitizer. Just like the food you put in your body and the products you clean your house with, it's important to look at the safety of the products you put on your body.

Many women apply more than 20 products a day! That's more than 5 pounds of toxins a year—and these get stored in your body's cells. The full effect of this accumulation of heavy metals and toxins isn't truly yet known.

Chemical body care actually disintegrates the connective tissues of skin cells. Let's repeat that: your skin actually *disintegrates* with the application of chemicals. And that's all in the name of beauty. The regimens that promise beautiful skin are actually creating blemishes, dry or patchy skin, sensitivity, and inflammatory issues. The vegetable oils that are polyunsaturated trans fats—like mazola, canola, corn, and soy—are made up of omega-6s and are horrific for skin cells. When we ingest distorted, artificial omega-6 fats, they get absorbed into our skin cells, predisposing us to premature wrinkles and other inflammatory issues. The health of our tissue is really what beauty is about and is the best indicator of age.

The Environmental Working Group (EWG) states that "On average, consumers use about 10 personal-care products containing 126 ingredients per day." Of these products, studies have found that cosmetic ingredients like phthalate plasticizers, paraben preservatives, the pesticide triclosan, synthetic musks, fragrances, and sunscreens are common pollutants.

On top of that, the U.S. Food and Drug Administration can't require companies to test products for safety. The EWG warns that studies show as many as half of the personal-care products on the market have at least one chemical linked to either reproductive problems or cancer.

Here are some more unsettling facts:

- 22 percent of all personal-care products may be contaminated with the cancer-causing ingredients.
- 60 percent of sunscreens contain the potential hormone disruptor oxybenzone that readily penetrates the skin.
- 61 percent of tested lipstick brands contain residues of lead.

So what are we to do? It can feel quite overwhelming to have to be so vigilant about the products we use. Start by taking it slowly! Do a bathroom cleanse! Get rid of the false promises and the quick fixes. Read the labels on your products in the same way you read them on your food.

What products are you using now? Use websites like ewg.org/skindeep to see if the products you use are safe and to help you navigate to better choices. Remember, this, like the Conscious Cleanse, is not an all-or-nothing proposition!

Following are some companies making products that are safe for our hair, teeth, skin, and bodies:

California Baby: great line for kids and infants

Dr. Alkaitis: skin care, shampoo, and body care for both women and men

Dr. Bronner's: good for soaps

After Glow: full makeup line and a great source for toxin-free mineral makeup

Hugo Natural: good find for body lotion, hand sanitizer, shampoo, and conditioner

Living Libations: overall great resource for toxin-free beauty care

No Miss: go-to for nail polish, nail polish remover, lip gloss, mascara, and eye makeup remover

Pangea Organics: great for skin care, body wash, and hand soap

Suki: makes a whole line of skin, hand, and body care products

Tom's of Maine: best for toothpastes, deodorants, and mouthwash

In Your Journal

How do you take care of yourself? How does it feel when you focus on taking care of your health?

Day 10: Perseverance Is Priceless

It's not that I'm so smart; it's just that I stay with problems longer.

—Albert Einstein

It's Day 10, which is *almost* Day 14, right? We notice in our programs that as we round the bend in Week 2, the drop-out rate skyrockets. Why is that? What is it in the mind that says, *Eh, I did pretty good,* or *I feel awesome now, so I must be good to go.* Do you recognize something about yourself in either of these statements? Do you feel as though you've been plugging along, barely surviving the process?

If this is you, *stop right now!* It's time to recalibrate. It's time to find ways to enjoy your life. It's time to take yourself on a date. Go out and eat a delicious meal that's cleanse-friendly. It's time to get together with your friends and family and laugh and have a good time. Just because you're cleansing doesn't mean you need to isolate yourself. This isn't about suffering!

Visualize your end result. Imagine the feeling of moving past the discomfort and seeing this process through to the very end. There's no need to "hang on tight" or "hang in there" because you are completely free. You hold the power here, and what awaits you in the second weekend of purification and the reintegration phase will change your life forever!

We know that's a big promise, and it's one we have no issue shouting from the rooftops. Shine on! You've got this!

Conscious Focus: Quieting Your Mind

According to our beloved and most treasured author and inspirational speaker, Dr. Wayne Dyer, the average person has more than 60,000 separate thoughts per day! We have no idea how something like that is counted, but regardless, we all know what it feels like. Perhaps we should be called human *thinkings* instead of human *beings*.

"Thinking too much" leads to all sorts of trouble—particularly stress and anxiety. We dwell on yesterday's interactions at the cost of moving forward. We stress about a future that's not yet here. We worry about things we can't do anything about. And even when we can do something about them, we don't, because we're too busy worrying. It can be utterly exhausting, and it literally *is* exhausting our bodies. Much research shows that stress is directly related to disease. And after all, what is *dis-ease* but the lack of ease?

Trying to eliminate stress can be pretty stressful in and of itself. So don't try to eliminate it! Stress is one of your body's natural responses. We all have it. And it isn't going anywhere anytime soon.

Instead, focus on honing your ability to *respond* to stress. Practice tools and techniques for managing its impact, and work on making it a *motivational* tool, as opposed to one that inhibits you.

One of the best ways to manage stress is to learn to quiet your mind. This could be through yoga, meditation, tai chi, walking or running, listening to the birds, sitting quietly, or any other physical activity that allows your mind to let go. As an ancient proverb says, "The silence between the notes makes the music."

Say Yes to Yoga

We suggest you find a yoga studio in your area. Practicing yoga teaches you the art of controlled breathing, which is the foundation of meditation—the art of quieting the mind. For those who haven't yet tried them, yoga and meditation may sound extreme, but they've become much more "accessible" recently, and they're actually now being commonly recommended by doctors, scientists, and therapists as a means of healing and prevention.

Today's Action Step: Sit and Be

Take time today to sit quietly for 15 minutes. Set a timer, close your eyes, sit up nice and tall (sit in a chair for more support), and allow yourself to watch the thoughts that come into your mind, one after the other, like waves crashing on the shore.

Observe your thoughts, and observe your reaction to those thoughts. In meditation, this is called "watching the watcher." You separate "yourself" from your thoughts, and observe them without judgment, as you might watch a child deep in a state of play. Notice the thought in front of you, and consciously let it go. Use the image of the ocean to send the thought back out to sea. Notice the recurring thoughts and the emotion or energy you attach to it. Breathe in. Breathe out.

Conscious Eating Meal Plan

These last days of the cleanse are where the magic really starts to happen. New habits are forming. They're not ingrained yet, but you're no longer in wholly new territory. You're no longer a tourist, but you're not yet a local. There's a reason we ask you to take your appreciation, your *consciousness*, to the next level here. Don't take your accomplishments for granted. Don't back off them. Meditate on this scrumptious meal plan for today, and stay present.

Begin the day:

Drink 1 quart warm lemon water.

Breakfast:

Drink 1 quart your choice green smoothie. Why not make it a Blueberry Blast Smoothie?

Lunch:

Eat a big green salad.
Or if you're feeling creative, try Nori Wraps with Tahini Dipping Sauce.

Today's snack ideas:

Snack on Sherpa Spinach Dip with flaxseed crackers.
Or indulge in Spicy Zucchini Chips.
A handful of frozen red grapes can also curb cravings.

Dinner:

A bowl of Hearty Vegetable Stew with a handful of flaxseed crackers rounds out this day nicely.

End the day:

Sip at least 8 ounces warm lemon water.

Ingredient of the Day: Apple Cider Vinegar

If you made the Nori Wraps today, you likely dunked them into a dip made with apple cider vinegar. Apple cider vinegar has some amazing researched benefits to help with conditions, such as:

- Diabetes—it lowers blood glucose levels.
- Cholesterol—it reduces cholesterol levels.
- Obesity—it promotes weight loss and gives a feeling of being full.
- Cancer—it kills or slows the growth of cancer cells.

These are some serious claims! What we know is that our health can be measured by the pH levels in our bodies. The more acidic a body is, the more disease can thrive. In general, you want your body more on the alkaline side of the scale than the acidic side. There's a sweet spot right in the middle. Aim for that.

Living in polluted cities, eating the standard American diet, and taking lots of medications puts your body in an acidic state. What we're doing in the Conscious Cleanse is eating foods that reduce inflammation and promote a more alkaline environment. Apple cider vinegar is one of those amazing foods that helps put us back into the alkaline zone. We love to use it in dressing, sauces, smoothies—and even straight up as a health shot.

Apple cider vinegar can also be used topically to help with dandruff; acne; dull hair; and muscle swelling, aches, and pains.

Quick Tip: Moving Meditation

For so many people, the idea of just sitting quietly for 15 minutes sounds like torture. We understand it can be challenging to quiet the mind. Our thoughts tend to gravitate toward the path of least resistance, dominated by whatever's in front of us, stifling us from the ability to gain a broader perspective.

Consider the guidance that follows to help you settle into a short meditation. There are many styles of meditation, so find one that works best for you. Remember that 3 minutes of quieting your mind today is a win! Try for 5 minutes tomorrow. And remember, too, it's called a meditation *practice* because it's something you don't perfect overnight.

One of the ways we love to prepare the body and mind for meditation is through movement—not shocking coming from two yoga teachers. So find a way to move for 5 minutes. Do some quick sun salutations, go for a brisk walk, or do 100 jumping jacks. After your burst of movement, go immediately to lying down on your back someplace quiet and comfortable. (This isn't the time to take a nap and check out, though!)

Start by tightening your feet and calves for 5 seconds and then release them. Tighten your feet, calves, legs, and butt, and release them. Move up your body until you've tightened from your feet to your head and face. Stay lying down or come back to a seated position. Now completely relax and be still. Breathe in, and breathe out. Set a timer for 15 minutes. You may be surprised at how quickly the time goes by.

In Your Journal

When you quiet your mind, what do you notice in the silence—the in-between spaces? What did you notice when you sat for 15 minutes? What came up for you?

Day 11:
All You Need Is Love

Twenty years from now you will be more dis-
appointed by the things you didn't do than by the
ones you did do. So throw off the bowlines. Sail
away from the safe harbor. Catch the trade winds
in your sails. Explore. Dream. Discover.

—Mark Twain

Oh boy, do we have some fun in store for you today! We're so incredibly passionate and jazzed up about today's topics that we're going to keep our introduction brief.

The layers of the onion are coming off, and guess what? So are your clothes! Today is about love. Self-love. Now that you're clean and green on the inside, having pampered yourself yesterday, it's time to go yet another layer deeper. Keep an open mind, explore, and discover what it means to truly nurture and love yourself—and the gorgeous body in which you walk this earth!

Conscious Focus: Get Naked!

When was the last time you took off all your clothes and stood in front of a full-length mirror? There's a good chance it's been a while, we're thinking. But stick with us for a moment. This simple exercise can be very revealing (excuse the pun!), even transformational.

As you stand in front of the mirror, naked as the day you came into this world, begin by just observing yourself from head to toe—this is the hard part—without judgment. What parts of your body do you love or appreciate the most? Do you have great calf muscles? How about curves or freckles? A collar-bone can be sexy when you take the time to appreciate it.

Next, notice and appreciate the strength of your body. Acknowledge all the amazing things it does for you on its own. Your lungs breathe for you and your heart beats for you, even while you sleep. For some of you, your body has even created another human life! What about your spine? Think of all the wonderful, miraculous things your spine does for you without you knowing it.

For so many of us, our aches, pains, wrinkles, and extra weight cause us to self-judge, to write ourselves off, and keep us from seeing who we truly are. Often it's not even the physical body causing us pain, but our life circumstances, yet we punish our body as a way of coping. Who would you be without your pain? Who would you be without your stories?

Only when you are able to look at yourself will you be able to see yourself for who you truly are. And only then will you be able to heal.

Today's Action Step: Appreciate Your Body

You already know what we're going to ask you to do, don't you? Strip down and take a good look at your beautiful, radiant body. Look closely and say out loud, "I am beautiful. I am perfect. I am sexy! And I love you!" And then shoot yourself a big kiss!

Remember this exercise. It will do more for you than any number on a scale ever could.

Conscious Eating Meal Plan

In this section, we share some sublime superfood options. Enjoy and notice the benefits these foods give you: extra energy, clarity, and pure satisfaction that comes with eating the best nature has to offer.

Begin the day:

Drink 1 quart warm lemon water.

Breakfast:

Drink 1 quart your choice green smoothie. The Superfood Smoothie packs a punch!

Lunch:

Eat a big green salad.
Or for something even easier, try the Chilled Cucumber Dill Soup.

Today's snack ideas:

Kalamata Olive Tapenade with celery sticks or Spicy Zucchini Chips sound good.

Better-Than-Yogurt Chia Pudding makes a great snack, too.

Or a handful of walnuts will do nicely.

Dinner:

Whip up some Turkey Lettuce Wraps—and make extra for a healthy snack tomorrow! Slice up a few more shiitake mushrooms to add an extra superfood punch!

Or if you're feeling like a veg-head, enjoy the Blue Arugula Salad.

End the day:

Sip at least 8 ounces warm lemon water.

Ingredient of the Day: Superfoods

We've mentioned superfoods in earlier chapters, and with good reason: we love superfoods! What are they, you ask? Well, superfoods are a class of the most potent, nutrient-packed, ultra-concentrated, deliciously satisfying foods on the planet.

Here's a short list:

- Bee pollen
- Blue-green algae
- Cacao
- Chia seeds
- Goji berries
- Hemp seeds
- Maca
- Medicinal mushrooms
- Sea vegetables
- Spirulina

Crazy for Cacao

Enjoy cacao post cleanse in lieu of chocolate, and you'll never look at chocolate the same again.

Superfoods are filled with antioxidants and minerals and have been proven to have some seriously noteworthy health benefits. Superfoods …

- Increase the vital life force (i.e., energy) of the body.
- Boost the immune system.
- Help detoxify and cleanse the body.
- Reduce inflammation.
- Enhance libido. (Yeah, baby!)
- Alkalize the body. (Bye-bye inflammation! Bye-bye disease!)

But that's just the tip of the superfood iceberg. For more information on superfoods, visit our website at consciouscleanse.com.

Quick Tip: Let the Sun Shine In

If you live in the northern hemisphere and it's winter time, chances are pretty good that you're vitamin D deficient. In fact, a study conducted by the University of Tennessee Health Science Center concluded that a resounding 87 percent of Americans are vitamin D deficient! Most of us spend our days inside working, covered in clothing from head to toe. And when it's warm enough to be outside, we slather cancer-causing toxic chemicals all over our bodies to "protect" us from the sun.

We've become terrified of the sun because of the risk of skin cancer. And while too much of anything is dangerous, we, like virtually all life on this planet, need the sun! This certainly isn't a suggestion to go outside and scorch yourself, but you do need to go catch some rays. Give yourself just 10 to 15 minutes in the middle of the day, when the best UVB rays are available. These rays actually convert the cholesterol on your skin into vitamin D.

If it's logistically difficult to get these prime-time, midday rays, you should explore vitamin D supplementation, especially during the winter. The Vitamin D Council recommends you take 5,000 IU vitamin D per day for 2 months and then get your vitamin D levels checked. The ideal level is between 60 to 70 ng/ml. You may find that you can forgo the vitamin D in the summer and supplement with vitamin D_3 just during the winter.

Why the fuss over vitamin D? Here are a few of the benefits of optimal levels of vitamin D:

- Decreased inflammation and chronic pain
- Weight loss
- Reduced stress and anxiety
- Restful sleep
- Cancer prevention
- Cardiovascular health
- Decreased blood pressure
- Protection from autoimmune conditions—arthritis, multiple sclerosis, fibromyalgia, etc.
- Diabetes prevention
- Improved mood

Doesn't it make you want to go outside right now? If you're looking for a good vitamin D_3 supplement, visit lifespa.com for a high-quality liquid version.

Vitamin D and the Flu

According to the Vitamin D Council, new research shows the link between vitamin D deficiency and elevated risks of flu.

In Your Journal

How do you feel when you say out loud to yourself "I love you"? Do you feel funny? Does it come out naturally? What does it bring up for you?

Day 12:
Conscious Creativity

When the soul wishes to experience something, she throws an image of the experience out before her and enters into her own image.

—Meister Eckhart

T.G.I.F. ... or not? We know many of you are ready to go out to eat with friends, have a glass of wine or two, and not think about it anymore! We get it. We call it "cleanse fatigue," and it's definitely a normal part of the process. And it seems to get louder with the thought of the upcoming weekend. But let us lovingly remind you that you are *so close* to finishing, so give yourself the gift of seeing it through! Dig deep, remember your intention, and take a look at what a fun activity we have planned for you today. It's perfect for a Friday night, so enlist your partner or call over a few friends. Wow them with some baked kale chips, and serve Green Lemon Juice in martini glasses.

This weekend you have another opportunity to take on conscious purification. This round, we encourage you to up the ante by trying all liquids! Yes, you read that correctly. Liquids—fresh squeezed juices, green smoothies, broths, and lots of water. Remember, this is optional. You can most certainly repeat what you did last weekend if that's more appropriate for you. Refer to the "Intermezzo: Purification Weekend Guidelines" chapter for the purification guidelines.

Conscious Focus: Expressing Your Creativity

Today is about being creative. Maybe you read that and think, *But I'm not a creative person!* As you know by now, we like to ask you to try turning your initial perception upside down, and today is no different.

We are *all* creative. Each one of us is a creator, responsible for creating our own reality. You can choose not to be a victim of your circumstances, whatever they may be, and instead be the boss of them. Try this on for size: say out loud, "I am a creative being, responsible for my own reality." Now say it again.

Self-expression comes in many forms. It's a way for each of us to be creative, to create the life we've always imagined. How do you express yourself and your creativity? Do you like to sing or play an instrument? Do you like to decorate? Do you love to dance? Are your clothes a way you could more fully express yourself? What about the journal you're keeping during the Conscious Cleanse? When you look for them, opportunities for creativity wait for you at every turn.

Conscious creativity has power. Ever made a dream board? This is where you sit on the floor, flip through magazines, and cut out images that speak to you or represent something you'd like to create, be, do, or have in your life. You can also do this digitally (and gather inspiration from others) on sites like Pinterest (pinterest.com).

For the more tech-savvy, consider making your own movie and publishing it to YouTube. Create the movie of your dream life by filming yourself, speaking in the present tense as if the day of your dreams has arrived. Fun!

Today's Action Step: Express Yourself

Do something creative today. Redecorate a room in your house. Dress up and get funky! Sing out loud. Make a dream board. Write poetry. Make someone a handmade card. Find a way to express yourself that lights you up.

As always, it's the action that matters—so no judgment!

Conscious Eating Meal Plan

Going along with the theme of conscious creativity, as you plan your meals for today, consider checking in with your intuition to be sure this is what your body is craving. Sometimes, as we allow our creative juices to flow, our hunger for food diminishes. Be the observer, and eat accordingly.

Begin the day:

Drink 1 quart warm lemon water.

Breakfast:

Drink 1 quart your choice green smoothie. Need an idea? Try the Hemptastic Smoothie.

Lunch:

Eat a big green salad sprinkled with shelled hemp seeds. May we recommend the Wakame Cucumber Salad?

Today's snack ideas:

Enjoy a leftover Turkey Lettuce Wrap from last night's dinner.

A Lucky Banana Smoothie also makes a great snack.

Or nosh on a handful of Brazil nuts.

Dinner:

Serve yourself a bowl of Red Chard and White Bean Soup. (Pop the leftovers in the freezer for a quick and healthy meal next week.)

Make It an Early Dinner

Be sure you have your last meal on Day 12 before 6 P.M. in preparation for conscious purification.

End the day:

Sip at least 8 ounces warm lemon water.

Ingredient of the Day: Hemp Seeds

The hemp plant produces an amazing superfood seed. Hemp seeds are a complete protein source and have more essential fatty acids than almost any other seed on the planet. The ratio of omega-3 to omega-6 fats is 3:1, which is the perfect balance.

Hemp seeds' complete protein and essential fatty acids make it a good alternative to fish, which is becoming more and more contaminated with mercury. Hemp seeds also have more than 20 trace minerals, which are vital for optimum health, along with zinc, magnesium, phosphorus, and vitamin E. Just 4 tablespoons hemp seeds contain 12 grams protein and 20 percent of your daily iron requirements. Try hemp seeds in your salads, salad dressings, and smoothies, or eat them plain by the spoonful!

Hemp seed oil can also be used topically. It's a great anti-inflammatory oil that helps with eczema. Be sure not to cook with hemp seed oil, however, because it has a low smoke point. Instead, add it to your hot meal *after* it has been cooked.

Keep 'Em Cool

To keep them fresh, store hemp seeds in the refrigerator.

Quick Tip: Keeping It "Basic"

Remember those little litmus paper strips you used in science class that would turn shades of blue, green, red, and pink depending on what you dipped them in? Those litmus papers were testing the pH of your mystery substance. pH tells you how "acidic" or "basic" something is. The pH scale runs from 0 to 14; anything under the 7 pH is acidic, and anything over 7 is basic or alkaline. Human blood typically fluctuates between 7.35 and 7.45.

When we eat foods like refined sugars, alcohol, grains, coffee, soda, cheese, meat, and processed foods, however, this level dips down into the more acidic zone. Conversely, when we eat amazingly alkaline foods like dark leafy greens, seaweed, sprouts, and raw and living foods, our bodies become more alkaline. You want a slightly more alkaline state. Consuming too many acid-forming foods puts your body in a constant quest for balance. When that happens, your body actually mines alkaline minerals from your bones!

Here are some signs and symptoms you might be too acidic:

- Tense muscles
- Stress headaches
- Anger or irritability
- Itchy skin
- Acne
- Chronic negative thoughts
- Addictions (coffee, cigarettes, alcohol, or drugs)

Does it make sense why purification is so important? You get to replenish your body and really put things back in balance this weekend. Smoothies and juices are chock-full of minerals, vitamins, and enzymes, all of which help with your body's rejuvenating processes.

Even more, the alkalizing properties of smoothies and fresh juices help neutralize the acid condition most of us suffer from, as well as help us release toxins. So drink up those dark leafy greens!

In Your Journal

What inspires you? How do you express yourself and your creativity? Write about the life of your dreams in the present tense as if it has already come to pass. Represent all the five senses in your description.

Day 13: A Clearing in the Forest

When inspired by some great purpose, some extra-ordinary project, all thoughts break their bounds. The mind transcends limitations, consciousness expands in every direction and we find ourselves in a new, great and wonderful world. Dormant forces, faculties and talents come alive, and we discover ourselves to be greater persons by far than we ever dreamed ourselves to be.

—Patanjali

Now that you're nearly a pro at purification, have you decided to take it up a notch with the liquids-only option we mentioned in Day 12's chapter? Liquid purification—that is when you consume only water, fresh juices, and vegetable broth—has been around as a method of deep healing since biblical times. It has been touted as a means for rejuvenating the body, mind, *and* spirit. So today we're going to take you on yet another journey inward with the hope of deepening your experience. Open yourself to the possibility that through this process, you'll discover new things about yourself and tap into strengths you didn't know you had—strengths you can carry with you for the rest of your life.

This is, as they say, the homestretch. So continue to trust the process and allow the purification to do the work.

Conscious Focus: Living Your Best Life

We're getting down to the core of the Conscious Cleanse, so by now you likely have felt some significant physical changes. There's no more need for us to speak hypothetically—you already *know* the power of the nutritional cleanse.

But as we've already alluded, there's more to it than just that. Improving your symptoms, losing weight, getting out the pain—these are just the gateway to truly living your best life.

The average American sets some version of an intention, a resolution, or a goal at least one and a half times per year. And we all know how well those typically hold, right? The goal to lose weight, to quit smoking, to eat better, to exercise, to find a more fulfilling job, ... they don't stick because so often they don't take into account the greater meaning of a person's life. They're not attached to a larger purpose.

This is understandable. It's difficult to see the proverbial forest for the trees. Your weight; your addictions; your various aches, pains, illnesses, and disorders—that forest contains a lot of trees!

But look how far you've come in just a couple weeks. What you've given yourself is an opportunity: you've come to a clearing, a rise in the landscape of your life. This is a moment of clarity and perspective that not many people experience.

You've given yourself a gift. It can be a small one—a glimpse, a spark, a 2-week vacation you look back on and draw some inspiration from—or it can be something much, much more. Now is the time to attach meaning to what you've accomplished, to anchor it to a purpose.

It's impossible to make a resolution to live more joyfully, to live more energetically, to live a life of fulfillment. Where would you even start with a goal like that? But really, those things are at the heart of every resolution. We don't want to lose weight—we want to be released from the limitations that extra weight puts on us. We don't want to make more money—we want to feel more free.

Our resolutions tend to be nothing more than a means to some undefined ends. Now is your opportunity to define those ends, to give clarity and purpose to your actions, to take advantage of your accomplishments so those accomplishments become your new baseline, the foundation of your purpose-centered life.

Our wish for you this weekend is that you remember who you really are. You are more than your thighs; you are more than your job; you are more than the quantity of greens you consume in any given day.

Today's Action Step: Tune in and Listen

Sit somewhere quiet today and take a deep breath. Notice your body. Notice your breath. Do this for a few minutes and then place your hands over your heart. As you feel the breath move up into your hands and then into your heart, ask yourself, *What is my soul's deepest desire?* Wait and listen. Allow the answer to come from your heart instead of your head.

Sit quietly and reflect, or journal about the answers that come.

Conscious Eating Meal Plan

Today is a challenge. But you've come this far, which means you are strong in the face of challenges. Stay strong and forgiving of yourself. Today, like all days, is just 1 day. Surmount one, and use it to remind yourself you can surmount anything. Liquid purification is where your spirit rises to the surface. You are what you eat, but you are so much more.

Begin the day:

Drink 1 quart warm lemon water.

Breakfast:

Drink 1 quart your choice green smoothie (remember, ideally you'll avoid those with ingredients not included in the purification guidelines) plus ½ tablespoon your favorite oil. Need an idea? Try the Alkalizer Smoothie with ½ tablespoon hemp seed oil.

Want an extra-soothing boost? Add 2 ounces cold-pressed organic aloe to your morning smoothie.

Smoothie Suggestions

Remember to choose a smoothie without seeds, nut milks, or avocado. If the smoothie recipe calls for more than 2 tablespoons of oil, remember this is your oil for the entire day. We recommend you cut the recipe suggested amount to ½ to 1 tablespoon instead or omit the oil altogether and save it for later mealtimes.

Lunch:

Drink 1 quart your choice green smoothie (again, following the purification guidelines) and add ½ tablespoon oil. Need an idea? Try the Southern Bliss Smoothie without the flaxseeds.

We love sipping on 1 quart Fasting Tea to help curb the appetite and cleanse the body.

Today's snack ideas:

Sip some Green Lemon Juice.

Kick things up a bit with a Spicy Lemon Elixir.

Or opt for a Super Green Smoothie.

Dinner:

Try 1 batch Bieler's Broth drizzled with ½ to 1 tablespoon healthy oil of your choice.

End the day:

Sip at least 8 ounces warm lemon water

Ingredient of the Day: Aloe

When you think of aloe, you probably think of sunburns and the aloe plant your mom rubbed on your pink skin. Aloe is one of the best remedies for helping soothe the skin after it becomes inflamed from sunburn. But did you know you can actually drink aloe as well? Aloe has the same healing effect on the surfaces it's absorbed by internally as it does on your skin. When you drink aloe, it travels through your digestive pathway—mouth, throat, stomach, and digestive tract—healing everything it touches as it moves through your system. Aloe …

- Improves your immune system.
- Helps with digestive issues such as IBS, Crohn's, and damage from the standard American diet.
- Aids in safely eliminating toxicity from the body.
- Regulates blood sugar and helps lessen symptoms of diabetes.

- Increases the bioavailability of antioxidants found in foods and whole food supplements.
- Hydrates and moisturizes the skin, making it softer and smoother.
- Improves joint flexibility.
- Helps with chronic inflammation and pain.

We love using raw, organic aloe on our faces as a lotion. You won't need any other beauty products; your skin will drink it in and look radiant! (Be sure to opt for *cold-pressed organic* aloe if you want to try this, too. Visit herbalanswers.com for one of our favorite high-quality aloes.)

We don't offer any specific aloe-centric recipes in this book because the plant can be a bit pungent to taste, but it's nice to mix it in smoothies or a bit of fresh squeezed juice. Or if you're feeling adventurous, you can just shoot it!

Quick Tip: Nourishing Your Soul

As you approach round 2 of purification, you know from last weekend that you'll have extra time on your hands—time you normally spend eating or prepping meals. As your body is hard at work cleansing and detoxing, fill up your soul with these nourishing ideas:

1. Plant some flowers or start an herb garden.
2. Watch a classic movie.
3. Call a friend you haven't talked to in a while.
4. Go for a walk.
5. Light some candles, and take a bubble bath.
6. Read a good book.
7. Do some gentle yoga or stretching.
8. Start a gratitude journal.
9. Brew a pot of tea to sip and savor slowly.
10. Make love.

In Your Journal

What is your soul's deepest desire? What can you do today to nourish your soul?

Day 14:
Celebrate Your Life

Every blade of grass has its Angel that bends over
it and whispers, "Grow, grow."

—The Talmud

Congratulations! You are here! You made it to Day 14! How do you feel about that? Stop for a moment and really take it all in. Take a deep breath. Do you realize what you've done? You've dedicated yourself to your health and vitality for the last 2 weeks. Doesn't it feel good to give to yourself?

Recall now the intention you set at the beginning of the cleanse. Remember the conscious contract you signed in Part 1? Think back on your journey, about what it took for you to be fully present, to show up in spite of life happening, in spite of challenges, in spite of distractions and cravings. Give yourself a big heartfelt squeeze and acknowledge what you've accomplished. This is the time to focus on your wins, to celebrate every green smoothie and celery stick. To celebrate your willingness to make conscious, life-giving choices. This is the time to really celebrate yourself!

What we know for sure is that you are courageous. You are powerful. You create your own reality. You are in charge of your health and your life. You are your own healer!

Oh, and remember the wellness evaluation you did on Days 1 and 7? Be sure you fill it out again—and be ready to be wowed!

Celebrate You

What does *celebration* mean to you? How do you celebrate? Sure, there's cake or wine, but we want you to think about rewarding yourself in different ways. For the last 2 weeks, you've been learning how to nurture and celebrate yourself. What's worked? What's felt good? Consider rewarding yourself with a bubble bath, a deep-tissue massage, or a stroll in the park with a loved one. It only takes 3 weeks to develop a new habit—and this is a new habit to learn. You have 1 more week you'll spend reintroducing the foods you've kept off your plate during the Conscious Cleanse. Stay with your healthy glow. Know you can feel this way all the time, not just 2 weeks of the year.

Conscious Focus: A Vision of You in Perfect Health

The last day of purification is the perfect time to harness the clarity, openness, and self-love that have already put the wheels of transformation into motion. Lasting change is yours for the taking. You already know you are the creator, the maker of your own destiny, and it only makes sense for you to create a vision of yourself in perfect health.

This is much like the athlete who visualizes his or her race or performance before the actual competition. Research shows that athletes who practice visualization in conjunction with actual physical practice perform significantly better.

We've all heard the saying, "I'll believe it when I see it." But we want to suggest that it's actually the other way around. You have to see it (in your mind) to believe it! You have to see what you want for yourself and then begin to walk the path toward your own visualization. This may sound like setting a goal, but it goes much deeper than that. Here, your subconscious mind goes to work, and you self-actualize in the same way your heart beats while you sleep. Your mind is at work even when your body isn't.

Maybe this feels a little out of your comfort zone. That's okay. You've come this far. Humor us. This is a risk-free exercise. The worst thing that can happen is nothing at all. The best is nothing short of radical transformation.

Today's Action Step: Practice Visualization

Today you'll tap into the vision of your best health, your most radiant self. Find a quiet place to sit comfortably. Bring your book or your journal.

Before you begin, close your eyes and take a few deep breaths to slow down and get out of your head. Feel your breath move up into your chest. Place both hands on your chest, and take the next breath into your heart. Work from this place as we go through the visualization.

Breathe as you read this, trying to inhale for about five counts and exhale for five counts. Inhale through your nose, and exhale through your nose.

Now visualize yourself in a beautiful place where you feel safe and protected: by the crashing waves of the ocean, in a lush and fragrant garden, in the woods with a green canopy of trees above you, on a beach with sand in your toes and sun on your skin, … wherever your favorite place is.

Imagine there's a wise and loving person sitting in front of you. As you face this person, you realize he or she is *you*; this is your most radiant vibrant self, a vision of you in perfect health. Look deeply into your own eyes. What do you radiate? What do you look like? How do you feel? What is your heart's deepest desire?

Recognize that this person has the most profound wish for your happiness. This wiser you embodies wisdom and love. Imagine you are drawing the energy of this you into your heart. Your wiser self has a very important message for you. Tune in and listen.

As you hear the message, feel the smile come across your face. Feel its truth. Feel a sense of calm and peace. Take this picture with you, and know you can come back to it at any time.

Open your eyes and take a few minutes to write down what you saw. Write uncensored, letting the thoughts come to you in a stream of consciousness. The only one who needs to understand is you.

Conscious Eating Meal Plan

As you feast on these delicious liquid concoctions today, make it a point to savor each sip slowly. Your cells will thank you. Celebrate your accomplishment—it's a reflection of your extraordinary life.

Begin the day:

Drink 1 quart warm lemon water.

Breakfast:

Drink 1 quart your choice green smoothie, remembering the purification guidelines, plus ½ tablespoon your favorite oil. Need an idea? Try the Chard Love Affair Smoothie with ½ tablespoon hemp seed oil.

Smoothie Suggestions

Remember to choose a smoothie without seeds, nut milks, or avocado. If the smoothie recipe calls for more than 2 tablespoons oil, remember this is your oil for the entire day. We recommend you cut the recipe suggested amount to ½ to 1 tablespoon oil.

Lunch:

Drink 1 quart your choice green smoothie, or try a raw soup and add ½ tablespoon oil. A bowl of blended Raw Carrot Soup (keep the avocado out of this recipe to make it purification friendly) or Zesty Watermelon Gazpacho would hit the spot.

Need another idea? Try a Passion Parsley Smoothie.

Today's snack ideas:

Sip some ABC Juice.

Or kick things up a bit with a Spicy Lemon Elixir.

A Raspberry Creamsicle Smoothie would also hit the spot.

Dinner:

Eat 1 batch raw soup or enjoy a fresh vegetable juice. To begin to ease yourself off the cleanse, add 2 to 4 ounces protein (animal or vegetable) and an additional 1 or 2 tablespoons oil.

Need an idea? Try 1 batch Bieler's Broth sprinkled with sunflower seeds and drizzled with 1 tablespoon flaxseed oil.

End the day:

Sip at least 8 ounces warm lemon water.

Ingredient of the Day: Tea

We love tea! We love the flavor, the aroma, the ritual, the fresh little leaves, the art of brewing the perfect pot, the seemingly endless variety of choices, the health benefits—not to mention the cute teapots!

If your body no longer craves coffee, why go back to it? Try tea instead. The history of tea is as varied as its flavors. In most cases, tea was revered around the world for its medicinal and healing properties. And today in the United States, it seems the art and ritual of drinking fine tea is finally catching on.

Drinking premium, high-quality, fresh, loose-leaf tea versus tea from a tea bag can be likened to drinking an aged cabernet versus a $5 bottle from your supermarket. Fresh, loose-leaf tea provides more flavor, taste, aroma, and anti-oxidants than its more processed counterpart.

Tea contains natural cancer-fighting antioxidants. It's a rich source of vita-mins C and B$_6$, folic acid, and thiamine. It's rich in minerals, too, specifically manganese, potassium, and fluoride. In addition, tea has been touted for its role in prevention of cardiovascular disease. Maybe that's because it contains an amino acid that's been shown to reduce physical and mental stress.

According to United Kingdom Tea Council, more than 1,500 different variet-ies of tea exist, so why not start exploring?

Quick Tip: Finishing with Grace

We know there's often a hurried pace toward the end of the cleanse. Again, it's as if you've been holding your breath to the finish line, where a big exhale finally awaits. This, friends, is a recipe for disaster. If you've stayed true to the core concepts of the cleanse—that this is not an all-or-nothing plan, that it's not about being perfect—then you probably won't need the following tips. If, however, you're just biding time until the program is over so you can indulge your chocolate cravings, consider the following before you proceed.

Slow down!

- Take a deep breath, and say a word of thanks before your next meal.
- Take a media fast today—no computer, no email, no news, no Facebook, no TV.
- Light a candle or some incense while you prepare dinner.

- Sit in the sun this morning, and spend some time noticing the nature around you.
- Upon waking, stay in bed and with your eyes closed, take a few minutes to be grateful and to set your day's intention.

Change your mind-set!

- Embrace the idea that the cleanse doesn't actually end today. It ends a week from today.
- Commit to testing at least three foods in the later "The Reintroduction of Foods" chapter.
- Learn, live, and love the 80:20 rule, which we discuss in the later "Living the Conscious Cleanse" chapter.
- Realize that healthy living is not a hobby but a way of life.
- Affirm to yourself—and for yourself!—that you are worthy and deserving of a happy, balanced, vibrant life.

In Your Journal

What's the message you received from your higher self? What does this mean to you? What's your commitment for the reintroduction of foods part of the cleanse?

Part 3

The New You

Sustaining Your Positive Results

Success is not a place at which one arrives, but rather the spirit with which one undertakes and continues the journey.

—Alex Noble

You did it! You made it through the Conscious Cleanse! Step back for a minute and enjoy your well-deserved sense of accomplishment. Take stock of the way you feel, your renewed energy, and the weight—figurative as well as literal—you no longer carry. Look again at your Conscious Wellness Evaluation. You've come a long way in just 2 weeks. You've given yourself a hard-earned gift, and you're feeling great. We hope you're brimming with pride, because you've earned it.

The natural question now is: what's next? You're standing at another cross-roads on your journey. Which way you go is entirely up to you. You've proven to yourself that you're more powerful than your addictions, and false cravings no longer pull at you. You've learned to listen to your body, to feed it what it needs. And as a result, you feel better and you look better. The equation, although it so easily gets muddied, is really pretty simple after all: what you put in is directly related to what you get out. Seems pretty obvious once you're there, doesn't it?

The Conscious Cleanse is about teaching yourself to make informed decisions. It is about recognizing that every single action you take throughout the day is a choice, and that every choice has an outcome. If you simply revert to your old habits, you'll just as simply revert to your old way of feeling.

But that doesn't mean you have to follow a militaristic existence of deprivation to live your best life. On the contrary, balance is the key to fulfillment. And of course, as with any balancing act, success requires your attention. You've completed the *cleanse*, but you've got the rest of your life to stay *conscious*.

It's time to utilize the blank canvas you've created. Part 3 is, above all, about deepening your self-awareness, about understanding how *specific* foods affect you, so you can approach them mindfully as you move forward. When you make informed decisions, you tend to make decisions that are good for you. You can choose to eat the piece of pizza or the chocolate cake after you've weighed impulse versus outcome. Impulse will no longer win every time. You *choose* when it wins and when it doesn't. That's balance.

In Part 3's chapters, we help you build on the momentum you've forged, to integrate your new relationship with your body into your everyday life, to find your *balance*. Welcome to the rest of your vibrant life!

The Reintroduction of Foods

One of the very nicest things about life is the way
we must regularly stop whatever it is we are doing
and devote our attention to eating.

—Luciano Pavarotti

In this chapter, we show you how to begin bringing the foods you've kept off
your plate during the cleanse back into your diet again. We know you'll be
shocked to learn that we feel it's important to do this consciously and with
purpose.

We take you through the eye-opening process of food testing and discuss what
to do with the things you learn. So trust us here: *take it slow*. We know you're
excited to be through the cleanse. We know you probably can't wait to take
the first bite of those foods you've been missing. But the *way* you reintroduce
these foods is *crucial* to this process. We urge you not to blow off this chapter.
You've worked too hard over the last few weeks to not use the unique opportunity you've given yourself.

Starting Slowly

Consider this: right now, your body is clean, energized, and working optimally.
In this state, you'll know very quickly what foods make you feel good and what
foods could be sabotaging your health. So rather than diving in head first,
we're going to guide you through a process to isolate the various allergens
you've been avoiding so you can experience how each of them affects you
individually.

As we've mentioned before, many people with food sensitivities and allergies
are unaware of them, even when their reactions are relatively severe. We've
heard some version of it over and over again from our participants: "There's
no way I'm going to stop eating cheese," or "I can't live without bread," or

"Eggs define my morning, so I'd rather not know." But ignorance, in this case, is not bliss, and knowledge is power.

Inspirational poster clichés aside, we understand the apprehension associated with sensitivity-testing the foods you love. But with this new information, you get to choose what you eat in a new and powerful way. Your options are no less limited—they're just better informed.

So pat yourself on the back, but maybe not with a slice of Mississippi Mud Pie just yet. This is where you really start designing your own perfect diet—one that fits into your lifestyle and meets your individual tastes.

What's Slowing You Down?

If you're like many people in our programs, your first thought about food testing was, *This doesn't apply to me; I'm not allergic to anything.* But hold on a second. Allergies and sensitivities show up in more than just extreme and obvious symptoms like hives, rashes, itchy eyes, congestion, or runny nose. Your body exhibits many other reactions to food, such as:

- Acid reflux
- Anxiety, mood swings, depression, or behavioral problems
- Arthritis, joint pain, or back and muscle pain
- Asthma or difficulty breathing
- Bad breath
- Body aches and pains
- Body twitches
- Diarrhea, stomach aches, or stomach pains
- Dizziness
- Fatigue or drowsiness
- Headaches or brain fog
- Hyperactivity or restless feelings
- Insomnia or change in sleep patterns
- Itchy skin, rash, psoriasis, dandruff, or acne
- Low energy or fatigue
- Nausea or vomiting
- Puffy face or swelling

- Sluggish digestion, bloating, or constipation
- Water retention or weight gain

Think about even the subtle differences in the way you feel since you began the cleanse. There's a simple reason for those differences: you've fed yourself more of what your body needs and less of what slows it down. Food testing just helps you get more specific about those foods that slow you down. So keep an open mind. You're on the brink of even deeper self-discovery.

There are actually two types of allergies: fixed and unfixed. Fixed allergies are ones your body simply can't tolerate. Typically, people are born with these types of allergies, and when triggered, the allergies often result in a severe reaction. Unfixed allergies, or "sensitivities," are allergies to foods often consumed on a regular basis to which the body has become intolerant. We refer to a fixed reaction as an allergy and an unfixed reaction as a sensitivity.

Sensitivities can be especially problematic because the reactions they cause are often subtle or indirect enough that the effect is rarely, and sometimes never, linked to the cause. You sabotage your health without even knowing it.

And sensitivities to ubiquitous foods like gluten, dairy, soy, sugar, and corn really pile up. And it's not just when you eat an ear of corn on the cob—corn sugar, corn syrup, corn starch, corn oil, and even foods like beer and whiskey can add to your body's reaction, until one day you find yourself diagnosed with a "chronic" disorder.

Food Testing 101

Over the last 2 weeks, you've essentially eliminated all the major allergens from your diet. If you're feeling better—and we're pretty sure you are—odds are, your body is sensitive to one or some of the foods you've avoided while on the cleanse. But in the course of the standard American diet—where likely you'll consume most of, if not all, these allergens in a single day or even a single sitting—it's next to impossible to know what exactly is affecting you and how.

But right now, you have the unique opportunity to utilize your "clean slate." By reintroducing these allergens one by one, you'll be able to see how your body responds to each. This kind of food testing is not a science, but in many ways, it can be more accurate than even an allergy blood test.

When reintroducing foods, as with the cleanse itself, you are your own best advocate. You know how you feel more precisely than the best doctors ever could. This, of course, isn't to imply you shouldn't see doctors for your ailments. It's important to listen to what your body is telling you and trust that it knows what it needs. Your diet doesn't need to work for anyone but you.

Testing for Allergies and Sensitivities

So let's get started. You're probably wondering which food you should test first. Ultimately, it doesn't matter, but you might consider starting with the foods you crave the most. Don't get too excited! Unfortunately, that doesn't mean you can test with a cup of cookie dough ice cream (which contains gluten, dairy, *and* sugar!).

Instead, test a single food in its purest form. If you want to test dairy, for example, consider plain yogurt or unsweetened milk. For sugar, it's best to explore food that doesn't have any other allergens in it. If you're not afraid of a rush and subsequent crash, you can always go straight Mary Poppins and take a spoonful of the stuff. For gluten, pasta or bread can be good choices, although you'll need to read the ingredients and be sure to avoid yeast, eggs, and sugar, which can be challenging. Just keep it plain and simple for now, and most importantly, take it slow.

Here are some allergen-isolating foods you can test restoring to your diet:

- Corn: corn on the cob, corn meal, corn tortilla
- Dairy: milk, yogurt, butter
- Eggs: one of the easier ones—just have an egg!
- Gluten: wheat pasta, wheat crackers, cracked wheat, cream of wheat
- Peanuts: peanuts, peanut butter (no sugar, corn, or any other ingredients—just peanuts and salt)
- Soy: tofu, unsweetened soy milk, edamame
- Yeast: dried Fleishmann's or Red Star Baker's Yeast

Testing for Yeast Sensitivities

It's best to sprinkle baker's yeast on some veggies or eat a spoonful to really test it in its purest form. If you find that you're sensitive to yeast, be sure you learn about other foods that contain yeast, too, like beer, wine, cheese, baked goods, some supplements, condiments, and soups.

Here's how to test:

1. Choose a simple food (only one allergen at a time) to test for the entire day.

2. Introduce the food with your normal cleanse breakfast.

3. Notice if you have an immediate response, including an increased heart rate, stomach issues, or any other symptoms, severe or otherwise.

4. Be conscious of responses throughout the day, including lethargy, bloating, joint aches and pains, etc.

5. If you experience no reaction at breakfast, repeat the steps for lunch and dinner with the same simple food you chose for the day. If you have a strong reaction, stop eating that food immediately.

6. Record any symptoms or observations you experienced on your allergy tracking form.

Allergy/Sensitivity Tracking Form

It's helpful to keep track of your body's responses as you reintroduce new foods into your diet. Tracking responses, like journaling during the cleanse, forces you to really pay attention to what your body is telling you and offers feedback you can analyze for yourself.

The following chart shows an example of what your tracking form might look like. Note that in this sample, we waited 1 day between some foods and 2 days between others. (More on taking days off from testing coming up in the next section.)

It's important to take stock of how you feel both physically and emotionally. Try taking your pulse. How did you sleep? How are your sinuses? There's no right or wrong way to do this as long as you're using the process to access information about yourself.

Use this form whether you plan on testing one food or an entire list of foods. You can download a blank Allergy Tracking Form from our website at consciouscleanse.com.

Sample Allergy Tracking Form

	Food	Breakfast Observations	Lunch Observations	Dinner Observations
Day 1	Cream of wheat	Ugh, gassy and bloated. Feel a little headache coming on. Foggy.	Ate cream of wheat again with lunch. Feel sluggish and tired. Still bloated. Haven't pooped—constipated?	Ate wheat again. Pretty sure I'm sensitive to wheat. Still haven't pooped. Gassy, bloated. Tired, lethargic.
Day 2	No food testing	Definitely allergic to wheat. Taking the day off. Still constipated. Ugh!	No energy, feeling irritable. Craving something sweet, need a pick-me-up. Drinking lots of water.	Small, hard bowel movement. Head still a bit foggy. Totally bloated. My stomach is sticking out.
Day 3	No food testing	Yeah, fog has lifted!	Finally had a good poop! Stomach not sticking out any more.	Feeling back to normal. No more gluten for me!
Day 4	Whole cow's milk	Drank ½ cup of milk with breakfast. No noticeable change.	Drank another cup. Noticing I have to clear my throat a bunch. Nose feels a little stuffed up.	Drank another cup. Again having to clear throat but not bad. Nose is runny now. My breath stinks.
Day 5	No food testing	Woke up really congested today, nose stuffed up. Taking day off to be sure milk gets out of my system.	I might have a slight sensitivity to dairy. I can probably enjoy dairy once in a while and just deal with the sinus congestion. This might be hard because I love cheese.	Feeling good! Sinuses are clear. Have a little diarrhea.
Day 6	Pure sugar	Put 1 TB. sugar on my morning cleanse porridge. Totally crashed 30 minutes later. Need a nap.	Added 1 TB. to afternoon tea. Felt anxious and irritable for about 1 hour later. Ugh.	Having massive chocolate craving. Not testing again. Feel icky, scattered, moody, no energy, lethargic.
Day 7	No food testing	Didn't sleep well last night. Feel a bit hung over today. No testing today.	Green drink for lunch. Seems to help me come out of the fog. Natural pick-me-up.	Starting to feel better. Not quite back to cleanse energy levels. Mood is better.

Testing Tips

It's important that you wait at least 1 day, but ideally 2 days, between testing foods, especially if you're dealing with any health challenges, are overweight, or suspect a food allergy or sensitivity. So if you test a food on Monday (Day 1), for example, wait to test a new food on Thursday (Day 4). On your off days (Days 2 and 3), return to your normal Conscious Cleanse eating.

It can take 3 or 4 days to eliminate an allergen from your system, so if you have a severe response, give yourself some extra time before testing a new food. Return to Conscious Cleanse eating during this time.

If you have a severe allergic response, be sure to flush your system with lots of water.

When it comes to listening to your body's reactions, sweat the small stuff. Even if the reaction you experience isn't on the list we gave you earlier in this chapter, consider what feedback your body is giving you. Stay curious about your responses. For example, we've seen participants get angry or aggressive after eating sugar.

For a more quantitative result, experiment with how your heartbeat changes after eating a certain food. Take your resting pulse before you eat the food you're testing and then again 20 minutes after you eat. Don't get too hung up on numbers; just use this as another way to tap into your body's messaging.

Taking Your Resting Pulse

A normal resting heart rate ranges from 60 to 100 beats per minute. To find yours, when you're calm and haven't just exerted yourself, grab a stopwatch or a watch with a second hand. Find your pulse, either on your wrist or on the side of your neck just under your jaw, using your index finger and middle finger together (not your thumb because it carries a pulse of its own). Count how many beats occur within 60 seconds. Or count the beats in 10 seconds and multiply that number by 6. If you count 11 beats in 10 seconds, your resting pulse is 11 × 6, or 66 beats per minute. If you have a heart rate monitor, you can also use it.

You may experience a more severe response to a food you didn't think was a problem before. That's normal. Now that you're a clean and green machine, your body is more responsive and sensitive than it was before you started the cleanse.

If you test a food in the morning and experience a reaction, don't test that food again for lunch or dinner. Stop eating that food immediately—you've got the information you need, so no need to suffer further.

How to Use Your Results

The foods you are sensitive to also make you gain weight. Allergens cause inflammation. Inflammation interferes with your body's ability to properly digest food and causes you to hold on to weight.

As we've said throughout the book, it's not about calories. It's about the *types* of food you put into your body. As you continue to reduce your exposure to the foods you're sensitive to, the pounds will continue to melt away.

The Puffy Factor

Maybe you've experienced the frustration of puffiness. You look in the mirror in the morning and either feel good about yourself or deflated based on the puffiness of your face. Literally overnight, you look like you've gained weight, and you feel like you have no control over it. It should come as no surprise to you now that the puffiness is your body's response to allergens. When you're inflamed and toxic, you retain water, which makes you look puffy. Even though you're drinking more water now, you retain less. Remove the allergens, and you lose the puffy factor.

Consider this: do the foods you crave taste better than the feeling of vibrant health? Do those fleeting moments of short-term satisfaction outweigh you living your best life? It may seem extreme to think about eating a clean diet 24/7, but shift that perspective for a minute. Does it seem extreme to look and feel good all the time? We think not. Once again, it comes down to finding your balance. We explore this a little more specifically in the next chapter.

But before that, it's important that you *consciously* decide how you're going to move forward and commit to your plan in the same way you committed to the cleanse itself. You have some options on how to proceed from here.

Option 1: Stick with the Conscious Cleanse eating program. You may be feeling so good you're not ready for the program to be over. There's no one forcing you to stop! You can continue to eat this way all the time or for as long as you choose. And you'll continue to see amazing results!

Option 2: Use the week (or two) following the cleanse to test for allergies or sensitivities. With these results, you might decide to completely avoid the foods you're sensitive to, recognizing that increased energy, weight loss, positive outlook, stable moods, and other benefits are more important to you than eating that food.

Option 3: Use the week (or two) following the cleanse to test for allergies or sensitivities. Maybe you discover you're sensitive to foods you just can't bear permanently removing from your diet. You feel like it would be unrealistic to just stay away, like setting yourself up for failure. Maybe you'll consider a "rotating diet." Instead of eating this food every day, you rotate it in every 3 or 4 days or choose to eat it only once a week or enjoy it only on the weekends. This frees your system from a constant overload of foods it's sensitive to. Remember, when you're rotating in a food, you need to watch for that food in all its forms.

Conscious Success Story: Sustaining the Results

Bill was 45 years old when he first tried the Conscious Cleanse. He had been suffering from a mysterious "traveling joint pain" since his early 30s. The pain would affect one or two joints a night, primarily his knees, ankles, feet, wrists, or hands. The next day, the pain in that joint would completely disappear, only to affect another shortly after. The pain and inflammation were with him about 5 to 7 days a week. Nearly 10 years after he first experienced the symptoms, Bill was diagnosed with Crohn's disease after a colonoscopy. He began researching the disease extensively and came across an associated symptom called migrating arthritis, thus solving his decade-old mystery.

Since his diagnosis, Bill's doctors have been working with various combinations of drugs and dosage to try to home in on the combination that might help put his disease in remission. But when he started the Conscious Cleanse, Bill found that his joint pain disappeared completely. He also found that another symptom—soft stool—also improved.

Two months after the cleanse, Bill follows the principles about 70 percent of the time and is still completely pain free.

A Note on Varied Diets

It's important to mention that eating the same foods every day can create toxic buildup and ultimately sensitivities to that food, even if it has never been a problem before. So while eating oatmeal or eggs every single day may seem healthy, it can actually be a recipe for disaster.

This holds true even for our beloved green smoothies. It's very important to rotate the greens in your smoothies. You might be able to tolerate the same food over and over for a while, but in the long run, problems may develop. So although we're not by any means suggesting you obsess over never eating the same thing twice, in general, it's healthy to keep a varied diet even if you don't have food allergies or sensitivities. This is yet another secret to vibrant health.

So continue to be a detective and note the "healthy" ingredients in your diet. Notice if you consume them every day. For example, we've seen participants who drank almond milk, ate almonds, and used almond butter and almond meal every day. That's lots of almonds to be consuming on a daily basis. Unfortunately, you *can* have too much of a good thing!

Think about your grandmother's or mother's weekly meal plans: Monday, meatloaf; Tuesday, lasagna; Wednesday, fish; and so on. Upgrade the food choices, but utilize the wisdom of rotation. This ensures you don't create a new sensitivity for yourself and allows you to enjoy and benefit from these foods for many years to come.

Living the Conscious Cleanse

We come into this world head first and go out feet first; in between, it is all a matter of balance.

—Paul Boese

Here's something we never get tired of hearing: "I am going to eat this way for the rest of my life!" Those simple words actually make their way to us quite often, and for us, it's the most fulfilling sentence in the English language.

Our mission with the Conscious Cleanse is to help our participants create long-lasting, sustainable changes in their lives. By now you know we believe strongly that true change happens on a gradient—slowly, naturally, and almost invisibly, evolving on a gentle curve and adapting as necessary. We know this to be the secret to creating sustainable vibrancy.

We hope you have decided to venture into the art of food reintroduction so you can discover, without a shadow of a doubt, what foods make you feel the very best. Moving forward, you can use the information you gain, no matter how subtle it is, to inform your eating decisions and maintain the benefits you've achieved in the past 2 weeks.

We call this doing your ABCs—an acronym for "always be cleansing." This doesn't mean you should be on a formal cleanse year-round—far from it. But you can realistically eat and live in a way that supports detoxification and an optimal digestive system functionality *all the time*. Like a finely tuned engine, your body's systems should operate silently, behind the scenes, without you knowing about them. If you experience stomach gurgling, gas, abdominal pains, or irregular bowel movements, think of that as your engine knocking, and you'll know it's time to upgrade your fuel.

In this chapter, we discuss what we mean by "always be cleansing." We offer you, via a set of guiding principles, some simple concepts to support you in your ongoing pursuit of true health, energy, and vibrancy. Remain conscious of these principles, and you'll continue to move naturally toward your ideal weight, free of pain and other symptoms. Free, really, in so many ways.

Guiding Principle 1: Living the 80:20 "Rule"

Okay, as a general rule, we avoid the word *rule* because rules are made to be broken. But the 80:20 rule is the perfect exception to our nonrule rule because it follows one of our favorite sayings:

Everything in moderation, especially moderation.

The 80:20 rule is about following the Conscious Cleanse way about 80 percent of the time. The other 20? That's where you throw any notion of deprivation out the window.

Liberating, isn't it? Yeah, we love it, too. To sustain a lifelong path, you need to give yourself the freedom to stray from that path once in a while. You do this as a choice, and you do it from a place of empowerment, without guilt or regret, knowing exploration is crucial to the human spirit but that straying too far can get you lost.

So that piece of birthday cake? Yes! A glass of wine on Friday night? Yes! A burger and french fries? Yes! Biscuits and gravy? You betcha! As long as your sensitivities don't cause severe reactions, you can throw caution to the wind from time to time, knowing that it's you, in this case, who controls the wind.

Refining Your Sweet Tooth

As you continue down the path of conscious eating and dietary exploration, you'll find you can toy with your treats, making even your indulgences work for you. So when you *choose* to celebrate with something sweet or want to wow guests at your dinner party, know healthy, life-giving, nutrient-dense options can satisfy the call for dessert. We have a selection of recipes for wonderful, super-good superfood alternatives to get you started in Part 4, or you can visit consciouscleanse.com.

For simplicity's sake, this may look like sticking to the Conscious Cleanse principles during 5 or 6 specific days of the week. We've had a number of participants find success in keeping consciously clean during the week and then letting it go over the weekend. Others give themselves about four meals each week to stray. Of course, if you have a strong sensitivity to a particular food, you might leave that off your plate even when you're letting go. Ultimately, it doesn't really matter how you choose to break up your 20 percent, as long as you do it consciously.

During your clean time, you'll fix meals with the easy in, easy out guidelines in mind. Green smoothies will continue to be a staple of your day. And your diet will consist mostly of fresh or lightly steamed vegetables; some fruits; some nongluten grains; and some lean, organic, grass-fed animal protein or vegetable protein. It's also good to make mention again of the "food demons" we discussed in Part 1. Hopefully, it will come as no surprise that you'll want to continue to keep them off your plate when you're in the 80 percent zone. But as long as you're not having severe reactions, just about anything goes during your 20 percent time without running the risk of overloading the body and its detoxification system.

You'll find that a funny thing happens as you follow the 80:20. If you pay attention to it, you'll notice that even the way you crave things changes. All of a sudden, the "bad stuff" doesn't taste as good as you remember. Indulgences become more refined, and you don't need to "pull yourself back" the way you used to.

Many of our participants have described how they actually find themselves looking forward to their 80 percent as much as they look forward to their 20 percent. Balance is a beautiful thing indeed.

Conscious Success Story: Finding Balance

John is a relatively healthy, physically active past participant in his late 30s who describes himself as an "all-or-nothing" kind of guy. "When I'm 'being good,' I have no trouble being good," he says, "so I was never worried that I couldn't maintain the cleanse program itself—I was worried that once it was over, I'd find myself on another bender, racing to undo any progress I'd made." The cycle had repeated itself multiple times in John's adult life—the familiar roller coaster of steep weight loss curves followed by equally steep gains.

"I'd do well on some sort of strict regimen, reward myself for doing well by bingeing like I was being paid for it, then spend a month or two planning my next dietary scheme while eating anything that even remotely looked like food. I told myself it was okay because I was getting consistent exercise throughout, but every year I ended up with a net gain, and every year I felt just marginally worse physically than I had the year before."

John's wife turned him on to the Conscious Cleanse, and they participated in the program together.

"Something finally clicked for me," he says. "First of all, I lost weight (over ten pounds in the two weeks), my seasonal hay fever never showed up that year, and the sleep apnea that I'd begun experiencing completely went away. But it was more than that. The biggest difference was that the Conscious Cleanse itself felt oddly *easy*. Kind of like I was cheating. I'd changed the way I was eating pretty drastically, but I never had to fight, never had to use will-power, and I felt just ... great.

"When Jo and Jules talked about the 80:20 rule, something finally gelled for me," he continues. "I decided that I would stick to the cleanse during the week, and just let it go on the weekend. It made it much easier to go to business lunches or out with friends during the week and pass on things I otherwise wouldn't have, knowing that I could give in to that craving in just a few days, knowing that I'd let myself devour a loaf of bread or a pint of ice cream on Saturday if I still wanted it then.

"Some weekends I took advantage of that lack of restriction, some I didn't, but what I found was that I looked forward to being 'clean' as much as or more than I looked forward to being 'bad.' It's like that old philosophy that good can't exist without evil—I need both extremes, but now I feel like I have the 'evil' contained and under control. It gets put away at a specified hour (Monday morning) and I can maintain five days of 'good.'

"It's been over a year, and my doctor was amazed at my last physical. My cholesterol is significantly lower and not only have I kept off the weight I've lost, but every couple of weeks another pound seems to fall off. Most importantly, I feel like I've found myself a lifestyle that's manageable and natural."

Guiding Principle 2: Be a Green Machine

This principle is about keeping the dark, leafy green stuff at the center of your food universe. We swear by dark leafy greens because they're among the most nutrient-dense foods on the planet, offering all the good stuff with the least amount of collateral damage (waste, calories, toxins, etc.).

Most simply, this is achieved with the green smoothie ritual. Just add water, greens, and fruit; blend; drink; and be on your way. What a simple and delicious way to supercharge your body every single day!

Not a fan of the green smoothie? If you just can't make the texture or taste work for you, we suggest making it a personal rule of thumb to have at least one big green raw salad per day instead.

Load your smoothies and/or salads with greens like arugula, spinach, kale, romaine, watercress, collards, Swiss chard, dandelion, beet greens, and mustard greens. Remember the darker the leaf, the better the benefits. Sea vegetables are considered a leafy green on the superfood list and are one of our favorite additions to salads, but you can also find them in powdered form perfect for adding to smoothies.

A smoothie a day has what we call a "compound effect" on your body's health. Think of it as an investment into your body's health savings account. With compounded interest, the little bit you deposit every day is multiplied exponentially.

In his book *The Compound Effect*, Darren Hardy offers the formula for success:

Smart, small choices + Consistency + Time = *Radical difference*

We just love that. And here are some of the reasons why the smart, small choice of keeping a green smoothie in your daily regimen will ultimately add up to a radical difference for you: raw greens alkalize and purify the blood; strengthen the immune system; are high in the type of fiber that aids digestion; are packed with minerals, vitamins, and phytonutrients; promote healthy intestinal flora; may help reduce your risk of cancer; improve circulation; and improve respiration.

We love and cherish our green smoothies and salads for all these benefits, but perhaps the most important reason to focus on one big green smoothie or salad per day is that the regimen will naturally crowd out the other convenience foods that don't make you feel as bright. Without giving it much thought, you get satisfied by the good stuff, which in turn satiates the urge for the other not-as-good stuff.

Guiding Principle 3: Eat in Good Food Combinations

As you've probably noticed by now, the guiding principles offered in this chapter are also the crucial components of the Conscious Cleanse. That's no coincidence.

Eating in easy in, easy out food combinations works in "real life" as well as it works on the cleanse. Following this principle 80 percent of the time is one way to ensure that your trash gets taken out every day as opposed to piling up and reentering your bloodstream, causing constipation, migraines, joint pain, depression, PMS, acne, fatigue, and many other physical ailments. No thank you.

Stay clean and clear by exploring the food testing strategies outlined in the preceding chapter to see whether certain food combinations work for you. This means more than just being gas free. If a food combination works well for you, not only will your digestive system *not* be talking back to you, you'll continue to lose extra weight (or maintain a healthy weight), have lots of energy, and see a general enhancing of the benefits you saw at the end of the cleanse.

While our focus during the Conscious Cleanse is about easy in, easy out food combinations, there are also a few other things to consider as you begin to incorporate other foods back into your diet.

Nonstarchy Vegetables

During the Conscious Cleanse, we focus on *nonstarchy* vegetables. But what about starchy vegetables? In general, starchy vegetables tend to require more time to be broken down, processed, and assimilated in the digestive system. But who can resist a baked sweet potato when it's cold outside, or a butternut squash in the fall?

We talk more about eating in sync with the seasons shortly, but for now, remember the basics of food combining with this exception: starchy vegetables combine with other starches (and of course, other vegetables!). That means they tend to work with whole grains like brown rice and quinoa, avocado (yes, it's actually a starch), legumes, and pasta. It's always best to combine your starchy vegetables with greens! So enjoy your sweet potato over a bed of arugula, for example, sprinkled with some quinoa and black beans if you like. Yum!

Beans—Protein or Starch?

Rice and beans are considered a perfect food combination in many cultures. So why is it that we don't combine them during the cleanse? This is a great question—and one we ourselves asked when we first learned to keep protein and starch separate in the stomach.

Beans, as we've mentioned, are uniquely considered both a starch and a protein. In the conscious eating guidelines, we treat beans like a protein because they provide an excellent alternative to soy and eggs. But beans also combine like a starch. So when it comes to your legumes, you really can have it either way: stay the course of the Conscious Cleanse, or enjoy them with brown rice or quinoa. Beans, like starchy vegetables, also combine perfectly with vegetables.

As with all food combining principles, remember that you are the ultimate rule-maker and the ultimate rule-breaker. Try some of the more subtle food combinations, and see for yourself how they work for you. The more clean you become on the inside, the more you'll pick up on the nuances of proper food combining. Likewise, the more enzymes you have in your digestive system, the more you'll be able to tolerate the occasional imperfectly combined meal. (Revisit the "Guiding Principle 1: Living the 80:20 'Rule'" section if you need to.)

Guiding Principle 4: Focus on Nutrient Density

Consider the following questions before you put anything in your mouth:

Is this the most nutrient-dense food I can eat right now?
Will this food make me feel brighter?

If the answer to the first question is "yes," then invariably the same answer will work for the second question. Nutrient-dense food allows you to take in the good stuff with a leave-no-trace effect on your body. When you consume nutrient-dense foods, you're left naturally satisfied because your body recognizes the intake of essential vitamins, minerals, trace minerals, antioxidants, and phytonutrients and knows how to utilize them optimally.

Consider, for example, clinical researcher and health advocate Dr. Neal Barnard's theory that when a human being consumes too much dairy, his or her body becomes confused. In an attempt to deal with the excess calcium, according to Barnard, the body actually steals from its vitamin D stores to process the calcium. So instead of being nourished by this food choice, a slight deficit occurs. These types of decisions, made consistently, add up and are influenced by the compound effect, only in reverse.

On the bright side, nutrient-dense foods—those whole foods available in their natural state—are some of the healthiest foods in the world. By now, you know the importance of whole food nutrition, but it bears repeating. Continue to fill your grocery cart with the package-free, colorful abundance of fruits, nuts, seeds, vegetables, sprouts, beans, lean meats, fish, oils, herbs, spices, and superfoods you enjoyed during the cleanse. Focus on foods that taste good and are readily available.

That brings us to an important topic: eating locally and seasonally. Whenever possible, it's a great practice—and highly educational—to focus on consuming food grown in and around your community. The average meal travels 1,500 miles before actually reaching your plate. That means a lot of your food is picked before its prime. When you eat food from your local farmers' market, not only are you supporting your local economy, you're also eating the freshest, ripest, most nutrient-dense food possible. Not to mention you'll be connected to your food at a deeper level.

Fresh Food on Your Table

Finding fresh, nutrient-dense food is easier than you might think. You can visit a local farm, sign up for a farm-fresh organic produce delivery service, or join a CSA (Community Supported Agriculture) in your area. If you're more of a DIY-er, you can plant a windowsill herb garden, start a larger garden in your backyard, or even get a plot in your community garden. You could also join the urban farm movement, or start a slow food movement chapter in your area. Visit slowfood.com to learn more.

The other great thing about eating locally is that you'll also be naturally eating more seasonally. Eating in tune with the seasons, aside from being more cost effective, supports your body's natural instincts. During the long, hot days of summer, we naturally crave light and cooling foods like fruits and vegetables. In the cold and dark winter months, we crave more comforting, warming, high-protein foods, like soups, meat, nuts, and seeds. And in the spring when everything is fresh and new, we move toward leafy green salads, berries, and fresh herbs. As you tune in to your body, it's only natural that you'll begin to tune in to your environment. Looking to nature is always a great way to stay on the right track.

Lastly, we'd be remiss in discussing nutrient density without mentioning superfoods. Superfoods can help ensure you get the full spectrum of vitamins and minerals. This is a food world in and of itself, so explore superfoods slowly, and don't be afraid of trying new things. Some of our favorite superfoods are cacao (raw chocolate beans, when not cleansing), chia seeds, maca, hemp seeds, and sea vegetables. Check out sunfood.com, or ask your local health food market to steer you in the right direction when it comes to superfoods.

Guiding Principle 5: Keep Your Soul Food Balanced

This last principle may seem a little less specifically instructive—and it is—but everything in the Conscious Cleanse, really, leads to this.

As humans, we yearn to feel good physically because when we do, we are free to focus beyond our physical selves, and we move toward true fulfillment. Food is the bodily fuel that allows us to feed our souls and satisfy an innate desire for a happy and fulfilling life.

Remember every day how much more you are than the things that pull at you: the size of your thighs, your job, your health concerns, your carpool schedule, your household responsibilities, your life's challenges, and all the stories you tell yourself. Physically, you are what you eat. Spiritually, you are so very much more. In the end, you take care of your body because it houses your soul.

On a long international flight, a plane flies off course 90 percent of the time. The pilot's job, with the help of the onboard navigation systems, is to constantly correct course so the plane ends up as scheduled in Los Angeles as opposed to Cancun. You are the pilot of your life. You man the controls. So how can you keep your course corrected toward your best and most vibrant life?

Consider the following exercise. Rate yourself in each one of the soul food categories, and ask yourself, *If this were the wheel of my life, would it be balanced? Would I be rolling along smoothly?* If the answer is "no," consider how you can give yourself a tune-up by paying some more attention to those unbalanced areas of your life.

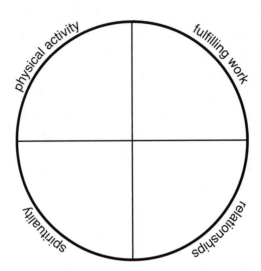

Your soul food chart—how balanced are you?

Consider each area of soul food in your life. Starting from the center of the circle, shade each quarter to represent how satisfied you are in this area. The larger the slice, the more satisfied you are with this aspect of your life.

How balanced is your circle? How balanced is your life? What can you do today to bring even a little balance to that area of your life?

Treat yourself gently and kindly, as you would treat a small child. Pay attention to your needs. When you cleanse your body, you also cleanse your mind. You free yourself to rediscover your passions. Let your conscious eating be the string around your finger to help you remember *yourself.* Take action—big or small, it doesn't matter—to do something for *you* every day. Make that time. Feed your soul. That's the truest nourishment there is.

Troubleshooting Real-Life Distractions

Reality is that which, when you stop believing in it, doesn't go away.

—Philip K. Dick

Let's face it: life happens. The Conscious Cleanse doesn't suppose you're able to live every day at a fancy spa retreat. We all have daily responsibilities and social lives that aren't necessarily conducive to cleansing. This chapter helps you navigate some of the most common "distractions" you're likely to face while cleansing and on the road to optimal health.

Eating in Restaurants

Although we certainly don't suggest you eat every meal of the cleanse at a restaurant, dining out is often required for work, for special occasions, as a way to connect with friends, or just to fill the need to get out of the house from time to time.

While on the cleanse, or even after the cleanse, restaurants can feel a bit daunting. After all, most restaurants aren't in the business of keeping food *off* your plate. The pull of the warm bread basket, the descriptions of pastas in cream sauces, and so much more can make you feel like you're missing out.

And although it's true that while cleansing you'll have to forgo the offered decadence, you can still enjoy much of the ritual of dining out. After all, someone prepares your food for you, brings it to you, and cleans up after you. Dining out allows you to really slow down and focus on the people you're with and savor your food without one eye on the sink full of pots and pans.

Like so much in the Conscious Cleanse, as in life, a little change in perspective can go a long way. Put on the lens of what you *can* eat, focus on really enjoying it, and suddenly you'll be wowed by your options.

Tips for Dining Out

Here are some tips we use when going out on the town:

Take a grab-bag of little add-ons to your meal with you—raw nuts, stevia, herbal tea, and a LÄRABAR, for example. You could even get adventurous, make your own dressing, and bring it in a to-go container. Don't be afraid to supplement with what you know will make your experience more comfortable.

Don't get caught hungry when you're out. Hunger will always win. The bread-basket, numerous fried appetizers, and other unsavory sides will be much less attractive if you aren't ravenous. Eat a handful of nuts or a banana before you make your way out on the town.

Ask for what you want. This is a great practice you can carry with you the rest of your life. Restaurants are in the people business. They need to please as broad a range of diners as they can, and they know satisfied customers come back. You might feel a little uncomfortable the first few times you order, but it gets easier—we promise! When we order, it sounds something like this:

> I've got a bit of a special request for you. Are you ready for it? *[Smile.]* I'd like the chicken Caesar salad please, without the croutons and cheese. What else is on the salad? Can you add extra broccoli, cucumbers, and olives? Thank you so much! Also, can I get olive oil and a few slices of lemon instead of the dressing? One more question, how do you prepare your chicken? Can you use olive oil instead of butter? I really appreciate your help. I know that was a mouthful.

Be playful and nice, and don't take yourself too seriously!

Finally, make your own dish out of the ingredients you see on the menu. For example, if you see a few sides of veggies that aren't in the same entrée, make your own entrée! Ask that the sides that sound delicious to you be combined on one plate as your meal. For example, you might have a side of sautéed kale or spinach and a side of steamed cumin carrots. Then just ask for some brown rice as well. *Voilà!*

Know Your Options

If possible, know them before you even get to the restaurant. These days, most restaurants post their menus on their websites and/or social media pages. Having an idea about what you plan on eating before you're tempted in a direction you don't want to go can be very helpful.

Here are some brief examples of "clean" options you might find on restaurant menus, starting with good drink options:

- Unsweetened herbal tea
- Sparkling water with a squeeze of lemon or lime
- Hot water with lemon

Sweet Success

Keep some stevia packets in your purse or bag, and use them to sweeten things up!

Here are some good appetizer options:

- Kale chips—some farm-to-table restaurants are serving them now!
- Grilled chicken skewers—ask for them without the sauce
- Hummus with carrot and celery sticks

And here are some entrée options you might try:

- Big salad with no dressing, cheese, or croutons—just veggies! Dress with olive oil, lemon, a dash of sea salt, and freshly ground pepper. Add some nuts, avocado, or animal protein on top.
- Steamed veggies with brown rice. This is a great choice at Chinese restaurants!
- Salmon without a sauce and a side of steamed veggies. (See what they have on the menu.) This is a great choice at fancier joints.
- Japanese mixed vegetable plate. Add a side salad and a fish entrée. This is a nice option when you're eating Japanese food.
- Chicken or veggie shish kabobs. Add brown rice if you're eating veggie-only kabobs.
- Chicken or veggie fajitas, hold the tortilla. Ask for a side of avocados, too. If the restaurant makes its own guacamole, they should have avocados on hand.
- Bison steak with a side of steamed vegetables and a side salad (no dressing, cheese, tomatoes, croutons, or fried onions).

Eating on the Road

There's never a *perfect* time to cleanse, so although we won't encourage you to start the cleanse before your next trip to Napa Valley's wine country, business trips and weekend excursions should not stop you from cleansing. In fact, we know a traveling salesperson who recently successfully completed the cleanse. With the proper preparation, she was able to be on the road, in and out of hotel rooms, for the bulk of the program. If someone with that type of schedule can do it, so can you!

As with every part of the Conscious Cleanse, traveling while cleansing is simple with the proper planning and preparation. Let's go over some tips to help you do just that.

Before You Leave

Scout out a local health food store and restaurants that offer a good variety of healthy options. We suggest going straight to the salad menu.

Reserve a hotel room with a mini-bar. Not an option? Be sure an ice machine is nearby. Consider packing a collapsible cooler—they're light and take up very little room—to handily store some perishables.

On the Road/in the Airport

Always, always, always pack at least a mini-version of a "conscious snack pack." Include an extra bottle of water (buy after you go through security at the airport), a baggie of nuts and seeds, and some fruit and veggies (an apple or pear, for example, and a baggie of carrot sticks). This emergency snack pack is simple but crucial. When hunger strikes and all that surrounds you are fast-food joints and convenience stores, you need a quick, healthy, satisfying option easily available.

You may want to consider bringing yourself a little "sussy," too—a little sweet surprise you save for special occasions, something to replace your old Junior Mints or Snicker's bar habit. A LÄRABAR makes a good sweet treat, as do dried mango slices or other dried fruit.

If you're driving, pack your conscious snack bag (or an even larger cooler if you have the room), with more food than you think you'll want for the trip. For example, blend a green smoothie and a raw soup, which are easy to drink while driving. Make a big salad topped with broiled salmon and a big batch of Quinoa Watercress Salad (not to be enjoyed at the same meal, of course).

A container of snap peas are great to pop when you just need that "pass-the-time" fix. You can store what you have left over from the drive in the hotel mini-bar for other meals or snacks.

At Your Destination

Make your first stop at the local health food store or market. Stock up on fresh fruit like apples, pears, and bananas. Buy baby carrots and a tub of hummus. Grab a jar of raw almond butter. Visit the bulk section and pick up some raw almonds and/or pumpkin seeds. Visit the deli and look for a simple chicken breast, a steamed veggie medley, and brown rice or quinoa. Don't forget to grab some napkins and utensils!

Bust out the ice bucket, load it with ice, and stick the most crucial items on ice—things like the hummus and the chicken breast. The other food will be okay at room temperature for a few hours.

Simple Meal Ideas

Remember, creativity is king. You don't have to stay within "breakfast food for breakfast, dinner food for dinner" limits. It's fine to have brown rice and veggies for breakfast. You don't even have to slice a cucumber—eat it like a pickle instead.

Another easy breakfast idea is to slather an apple and/or a banana with almond butter. Lunch can be as simple as baby carrots, cucumber, and hummus. Or go back to your health food store and order a fresh-squeezed green juice from the juice bar, or make your own green smoothie.

Eating During Holidays and Special Events

Contrary to what you might think, the holidays—especially the time between Thanksgiving and Christmas—can be an excellent time for the Conscious Cleanse. Nothing brings out our food demons like the holidays: the traditions, the sweets, the wine and spirits, the overeating, the indulgence, the lethargy. So while this might not be the first season you think of for keeping food off your plate, any amount of food consciousness during this time can have a profound and lasting effect on you.

Now, the thought of missing your favorite Thanksgiving dinner might sound like blasphemy, but remember, Thanksgiving dinner is just one meal. You can *choose* to indulge for that one meal and go back to the Conscious Cleanse for the rest of the holiday. It won't ruin your cleanse, as long as you get right back to Conscious Cleanse eating. The same goes for a birthday celebration, a wedding, or any other special event.

Being Someone's Guest

First things first: you are in charge of your own health—there's no reason to hide or be ashamed by that fact! As with the rest of the Conscious Cleanse, preparation and communication are key.

Jules is fond of telling the story of the proud and very sweet hostess who served her veal shortly after she'd given up eating meat. It's no fun to feel like you have to hide half your dinner under a garnish or sneak it to the family dog, so you're just setting yourself up for an awkward situation if you don't call ahead of time to let your host know about your restrictions. It can be as simple as explaining that you're doing a cleanse and you're going to have to be a little picky about what you eat. Maybe offer to bring a big salad or vegetable side dish you can eat and share with everyone else.

In the event it's not possible to call ahead or request a cleanse-friendly meal, be sure to start your day with warm water and lemon followed by at least a quart of green smoothie. Then, start the hosted meal with a big leafy green salad and strive to eat in good food combinations, even if it means you eat part of your meal in two sittings. For example, round one would be a big green salad with all the veggie and starchy sides available. Round two would be turkey and gravy. Skip the bread.

And why not bring your own dessert? Make some raw brownies or put a dark chocolate candy bar in your bag so you have a healthy alternative when the pie or the cake comes out. And if you bring enough to share, the hostess will probably appreciate the extra food.

Last but certainly not least, have fun! Don't take yourself or your cleanse too seriously! This is not about suffering or stressing over a piece of cheese or a glass of wine. Enjoy your food and your company.

Cleansing Amidst a Family of Noncleansers

In a perfect world, our children and spouses would eat what we eat ... and they would like it! Of course, the world isn't always perfect. It can be hard enough to get a toddler to eat a chicken nugget shaped like a cartoon character, much less spoon up a mostly liquid soup or chew a raw kale salad. And as adults, we can get pretty stuck in our ways.

Exposing your children—and often your partner—to some new tastes and textures can be a great strategy for creating healthy eaters with a varied palate in the long run, but it can also be disastrous—time consuming, emotionally draining, and wasteful. Trust us, you can't trick someone into doing the Conscious Cleanse. You can't make your husband an arugula salad and tell him it's mashed potatoes.

Remember that the goal is not to get the entire family on the cleanse—although that would be great! You might be surprised to find, however, they enjoy what you're eating and will be happy to share some of your fresh and healthy food because it tastes pretty good.

Enroll Your Family in Your Intention

Share with your family what you're committed to for the next few weeks and beyond. Be sure to speak only about yourself for now, regardless of whether your ultimate intentions include getting them healthier, too. It's very easy for people to feel threatened about their own food preferences when they hear about your work to improve your eating choices, so be clear that this is *your* journey and ask for their support.

It may be helpful to put in place a nonfood celebration to mark the end of the journey, something you can enjoy as a family, like a putt-putt golf outing, a movie, bowling, etc. Be sure to share your experience with your family, and be playful about the new foods and insights you're discovering along the way.

Don't Take Away; Add to the Good Stuff

Let's say your cleanse dinner is going to be an assortment of steamed veggies served over brown rice. Your family can also enjoy their pick of steamed veggies—if they prefer broccoli only, just include some more of it in your stir-fry—and a side of brown rice. If they're partial to meat, bake some chicken breast for their dinner, adding enough for your lunch the next day, and serve it to them on the side.

Most kids will love your morning green smoothies, although they may take some getting used to. If morning time is limited, make your smoothie together with them the night before. It will keep just fine in the refrigerator overnight.

Fun for Kids!

Get your kids involved in the smoothie-making process. Let them pull out the stool and stand next to you at the counter. As long as you're there with them, they can peel the banana, pour the coconut juice, and turn on the blender.

Start slowly by offering family members just a taste of a sweet smoothie, like one containing pineapple, banana, and romaine lettuce. Serve it with their regular breakfast, and pose it as a treat rather than as medicine. If your kids are older or if you're serving to a perhaps-petulant spouse and there's just no way a "salad" in a smoothie will be tolerated, get a little sneaky with a blueberry-based smoothie. This smoothie hides the green color and tastes even more delicious. Over time, you may find they're asking for more smoothie and less cereal or breakfast bar.

Stay focused on adding in the good stuff without taking away the food they're used to. If your children are used to eating mac 'n' cheese, for example, serve them a slightly smaller portion of the mac 'n' cheese, while adding some steamed broccoli and baked chicken.

Nobody will change overnight, and you shouldn't expect them to. Take it slowly. Focus on making better choices like brown rice pasta over the white pasta or sweet potatoes over white potatoes. Let them try your main course as their side dish. See what they'll tolerate, and see what they actually enjoy. Make this a part of your exploration.

Cook and Eat Together

Just as you involved your kids in making daily smoothies, include them in the grocery shopping and cooking, too. If posed correctly, it can seem like a fun activity and can help teach children about real food. Many kids (and adults, for that matter) don't know where their food comes from, they don't know the difference between a beet and a radish, and they've never heard of kale.

As you engage them in the process—not posed as a "have to" but as a "get to"—you can enjoy additional family time. And who knows, they might just become curious and want to broaden their horizons. Remember, in the beginning, a simple taste is a win.

Through this practice, one of our cleanse participants shared that she was surprised and delighted to learn that her kids (ages 3, 5, and 7) actually liked salad. When given the chance to eat what Mom and Dad ate, they were excited by the opportunity.

Another great strategy for creating a family of healthy eaters is to make it a practice to sit down as a family for dinner. There's something very powerful about a family who sits and eats together, without the distraction of the TV or anything else. This simple practice is a time to connect to one another, share stories, talk about your day, eat slowly, try new foods, laugh, and simply enjoy each other's company.

Cleansing on a Budget

There's no way around it: organic food at the grocery store is more expensive. We won't try to convince you otherwise. However, the money spent on healthy, organic whole foods pays back in huge dividends down the road.

We're strong believers that there needs to be a shift in the perception that food should be cheap, quick, and easy. We don't have room to really delve into this huge topic here, but suffice it to say, good, nutrient-dense, chemical-free, fully ripened food is more expensive to produce. The soils on organic farms are generally more nutrient-rich, so you get more essential vitamins, minerals, and trace minerals in your food. Many conventional farms have stripped the land of nutrients, and although the food looks the same, in reality, it might not be. Fewer nutrients, more toxic chemicals—not exactly what we're looking for in our salad, is it?

We believe toxin-free whole food is worth the investment. It's more expensive than conventional food, but less expensive than chronic health concerns. Organic practices are coming more into the mainstream, and with more availability comes cheaper pricing. Even Walmart has gotten into the organic game!

The following sections share some tips we've picked up for purchasing whole foods in the most cost-effective ways.

Plan Your Meals

There's that word again—*plan*. Knowing specifically what you're going to prepare helps prevent multiple trips to the market—and the associated impulse shopping—and prevents the food and money waste associated with "overshopping."

Be prepared for your week by scheduling your own meal plan, or follow our guidelines in the 14-day program. For example, making big batches of rice or sliced veggies is not only convenient, but it's also cost effective.

Buy in Bulk

Buying in bulk for things like nuts and nongluten grains can significantly bring down the cost of some of these staples. Your local market, as well as big-box wholesalers like Costco and Sam's Club offer bulk buying options, like frozen organic fruit, for example. You can also save on spices and herbs. Buy a glass storage container to store these items so they keep longer.

Make It Yourself

Skip the packaged foods when possible. The branded products will really run up your grocery bill.

Instead, make your own salad dressing, sauces, nut milks, and more! If you aren't a natural cook, this may sound daunting, but it's not as challenging as you might think. You'll learn something new and feel a real sense of accomplishment by taking part in your own food prep.

Buy Local

When shopping directly from the source, not only are you eating the freshest, most nutrient-dense foods available, but in cutting out the middleman, you'll also most likely be getting a good price.

For convenience, consider joining a CSA program (community supported agriculture; a simple web search can generally direct you to what's available in your area). Buy directly from your farmer at the farmers' market, or hire a company that delivers veggies to your door. These options all can be a lower cost.

Eat Less Meat

Meat is a more expensive grocery item, especially when you focus on grass-fed, organic meat. Shift away from meat at every meal, or even every day, and watch your grocery bill lower. Try an entire day without meat and see how you feel. You may surprise yourself!

Eat Seasonally

When food doesn't need to be shipped from long distances to places where it's currently out of season, the price goes down. Focusing on in-season food grown in your region helps bring down the bill and also works to differentiate your diet throughout the year—a great and important practice.

If you aren't sure what's in season in your area, use websites like Sustainable Table (sustainabletable.org) to find out what's available locally.

Another tip is to buy extra fruit in the summer and freeze it to enjoy all winter long!

Plant a Garden

Even if you don't consider yourself a green thumb, you might be surprised just how easy it can be to grow food on a small scale. Seeds are smart little buggers, and they're designed to flourish. A little sun, water, and a bit of TLC, and you're on your way! Start small, with easier, more robust crops like tomatoes and herbs. Think about the items you constantly buy at the store.

The same $5 you pay for a pound of produce buys you enough seeds to feed you for weeks. Many grocery stores even sell "starter" plants to help get you going.

Frequently Asked Questions

Better to ask twice than to lose your way once.
—Danish proverb

In this chapter, we've gathered some of the questions we hear most often from Conscious Cleanse participants in the hopes that something here might answer a question in your mind, too. For more, or to ask a question yourself, please visit our website at consciouscleanse.com.

Can I do the Conscious Cleanse while pregnant or nursing?

Most importantly, we always advise seeking the guidance of your health-care provider before beginning the Conscious Cleanse, and this would be no exception.

In general, it's not advisable for a pregnant or lactating woman to induce any type of detox because the body's reactions can affect the baby. That being said, the Conscious Cleanse—with the exception of the purification weekends—offers a very healthy way for pregnant and nursing women to eat! The key is to transition very slowly so you don't cause any drastic detox. Make any adjustments you need along the way. You may find you need to eat more food than you're used to, and that's fine.

When eating whole foods, weight should not be a concern, and whatever weight you gain during pregnancy, if based on nutritious choices, will effortlessly fall off after you have the baby.

Can I eat packaged foods if they're all natural and the ingredients don't fall into the "foods to keep off your plate" category, such as hummus?

Whenever possible, we recommend making things from scratch. This ensures you're consuming the highest-quality ingredients. At the same time, we know life gets busy and it's not always possible to prepare foods from scratch.

Don't just trust marketing claims on the front of the package. Examine labels. Seek out the brands with the fewest and cleanest ingredients, and avoid those with preservatives and ingredients you don't know or can't pronounce.

Does Odwalla or Naked Juice count as a "fresh juice"?

Sorry, but nope. These types of juices are marketed as fresh juices—and are certainly a healthier choice than diet soda—but they're mostly "fruit juice concentrate" (read: sugar) and pasteurized. What vitamins and minerals were in the product are greatly reduced in the process of pasteurization.

For a fresh juice, go to the juice bar where you see the whole food in its natural state (a whole carrot) and can watch it being juiced.

Can I drink kombucha?

Although there are many reported medicinal benefits of kombucha, it isn't something we recommend during the cleanse. Kombucha contains both sugar and yeast, and while it's suggested that the live cultures "eat it up," sugar is sugar, yeast is yeast, and the cleanse is a good time to take a break from both.

Do I need to buy only organic food?

We always advocate organic food whenever possible because of the toxic overload modern farming methods have on our food. However, we understand that this isn't always possible due to availability or budget. Check out the "Dirty Dozen" and the "Clean 15" at ewg.org/foodnews for the latest information on the foods that are most and least contaminated by pesticides, and shop accordingly.

Do I need any special equipment?

We recommend having a good knife, a decent blender, a cutting board, and a journal. If you have a juicer, a food processor, or a spiralizer, dust 'em off because you'll likely find new use for them during the Conscious Cleanse, although they're definitely not required.

I'm training for a race and/or I exercise a lot. Will I get enough food? And what about protein?

Yes, you'll get plenty of food! There's no calorie restriction with the Conscious Cleanse.

Good sources of protein on the cleanse include beans and legumes and organic, lean, grass-fed animal meats like chicken, turkey, lamb, wild game, and fish.

I have a lot of excess weight. What's my best plan of action?

Don't sweat it, and don't rush it! Stay the course and the weight will come off, consistently and naturally, until you reach your healthy ideal weight. If you want to keep the weight off, it's important, after your initially steep curve, to lose it slowly. The Conscious Cleanse is a great place to start! Follow the program guidelines, including the transition days and the plan for reintroduction of food. That, together with some mild exercise, and you'll be well on your way.

If you don't see the pounds coming off within the program's 2 weeks, consider continuing the program for 30 days, and follow the "Living the Conscious Cleanse" guidelines to support continued weight loss after that.

Discovering whether you have any food allergies or sensitivities will be a key factor in your finding your healthy weight.

I know I'm not allergic to a certain food. Do I have to give it up?

There are no "have-to"s in the Conscious Cleanse. That being said, especially if this is your first time doing the cleanse, we *strongly* suggest you try giving up that food for 2 weeks. After you're clean and green on the inside, and you systematically reintroduce the allergens, you'll know without a doubt how these foods affect you. Often it's a simple, subtle thing that won't mean you never eat a tomato again.

Remember, this is just about gathering information, allowing you to make powerful choices later.

How often should I cleanse?

Truly, the Conscious Cleanse, except for the purification days, is designed so you could safely eat this way year-round.

Generally, we recommend implementing the full program up to three times per year. We typically recommend cleansing during the first part of the year, to ride the wave of a new year, a fresh start, the feeling of rebirth. It's a powerful time of the year in our culture, so cleansing is often supported by the people around you. Spring and late summer are also excellent times to cleanse because of the abundance of fresh (and less expensive) produce available.

Strive to cleanse, at a minimum, at least once per year. You're worth it!

I've heard it's not good to cleanse during the winter. What should I do?

For many people, the thought of drinking a cold green smoothie is not apropos of a cold, winter morning, especially if you're used to a warm breakfast. When you have a strong digestive fire and a healthy metabolism, this becomes less of an issue.

Nonetheless, consider the warmer, more grounding options that are characteristic of winter. Opt for soups, stews, nuts, seeds, grains, and organic lean animal protein over the cold, raw food options. This is a part of eating seasonally.

Do you recommend I use any cleansing products in addition to the program?

It's not necessary to use any cleansing products or supplements to get the full benefit of the program. If you choose to use cleansing products, read all the ingredients and look specifically for a reputable, high-quality colon cleanse product.

For more information on supplements, please see Part 1 and visit consciouscleanse.com.

After reading about healthy colon function in the first chapter, I realize I'm not eliminating the recommended two or three times per day, or my stool hasn't really changed much from when I began the cleanse. What should I do?

Drink more water, and consider including more fresh green juices and fewer nuts, seeds, grains, and animal protein for a few days. Get some exercise. Massage your abdomen, moving from the right to the left side of your stomach. Take a hot Epsom bath—this will help relax your body and your digestive tract.

I haven't had a bowel movement in a day or two. What should I do?

If you've tried drinking more water and the tips we listed in the preceding question, you might take a more "hands-on" approach.

For example, one of our magic little bullets is 2 tablespoons of ground flaxseeds. This do-no-harm method adds an extra dose of nutrients. Add the seeds to your morning smoothie, and watch out, here it comes!

Add a high-quality magnesium to your diet. The most absorbable forms are magnesium citrate, glycinate, asparatate, and taurate. The recommended daily amount is 300 milligrams. Magnesium is a mineral that helps with stress and relaxation—and that includes your bowels! Some foods high in magnesium include sea vegetables, spinach, Swiss chard, and halibut.

Or try our herbal infusion, the Laxative Tea, or a store-bought tea like SmoothMove. We don't recommend other synthetic laxatives, as they can be habit-forming. Also know that herbal laxatives can be abused. Use it once or as needed, but not every day. Your digestive system is like a muscle, and when you use laxatives, your muscles don't "flex," so over time, they become weakened. Long term, laxatives can worsen digestive problems.

Consider a colonic or enema. You'll want to consider this approach based on your comfort level. Enemas may be more user-friendly for the novice cleanser. We also recommend, if you get a colonic, that you find someone who uses a gravity-fed system.

Your constipation can be an allergic response. You might be eating a food you're sensitive to. Is there a food you crave or notice you have a compulsion for? Notice if you're eating the same food or foods daily. Get more curious, and question everything you put into your mouth.

Part 4

The Conscious Cleanse Recipes

Making Healthy Food

A recipe has no soul. You, as the cook, must bring
soul to the recipe.

—Thomas Keller

In the following chapters, we present a collection of our favorite cleanse-
friendly recipes. On our quest for vibrancy, ideal body weight, and true
healing, we've tinkered with a countless number of them over the years,
gathering ideas from friends, cleanse participants, and experts along the way.
We're certainly not chefs by trade—just two girls who like to get creative in
the kitchen, experimenting when time permits and inspiration hits—which
is perhaps why we naturally gravitate toward simplicity. But you know what?
We've found that you don't have to be a trained culinarian to create extraordinary, satisfying, healthy meals. You just have to put together extraordinary,
satisfying, healthy ingredients and accept that not every experiment creates a
winner.

We hope these recipes take a little of the trial and error out of your Conscious
Cleanse experience. Don't be afraid to play with these recipes as you get more
comfortable. What follows are, after all, the winners that came out of our
many, many experiments. (As Julie says, "I've never met a recipe I didn't want
to change.")

More than anything, these recipes, like the journal prompts we offer during the cleanse, are meant to spark inspiration within you. Eating intuitively
begins with cooking and preparing food intuitively, so as you experiment
with these recipes, stay tuned in, trust yourself, experiment, be flexible and
courageous, and have fun. Making healthy food can be quick, easy, and exceptionally delicious.

We're always expanding our repertoire, too, so please feel free to share your
favorite recipes with us and visit our website and blog for more recipe ideas
and cleanse-friendly suggestions.

A Note on Serving Sizes

The Conscious Cleanse way of eating is based on the idea that when you clear out the clutter by feeding yourself natural, whole foods, your body intuitively knows how much it needs, so there's no reason to worry about overeating or compulsion. Everyone is different, so who are we to tell you how much you need to eat?

So during the cleanse, with the exception of protein and nongluten grain guidelines (generally try to keep protein—poultry, meat, and fish—intake to 4 to 8 ounces per meal and nongluten grain—brown rice, quinoa, etc.—intake to 1 or 2 cups per meal), we encourage you to listen to yourself: eat slowly and mindfully, eat when you're hungry, and don't eat when you're not. Don't be afraid to use leftovers for your next meal or snack. If a recipe doesn't look like it will provide enough food, feel free to increase it. And as always, have fun!

Green Smoothies

For years, we drank fruit, protein, and yogurt smoothies and thought we were being so healthy. And then we discovered green smoothies. By now you know what huge fans we are of these wonderful sippers. It's no overstatement to say these simple concoctions can completely revolutionize and transform your health.

Adding greens (the dark leafy kind, cucumbers, or even celery) to your smoothie amps up the nutrients, vitamins, minerals, enzymes, and fiber, and because it's liquid nutrition, they're easy on your digestive system.

For fantastic green smoothies, blend all the ingredients with 1 or 2 cups pure filtered water in a high-speed blender. You can add more or less water depending on the consistency you like. The less water you use, the more puddinglike the smoothie will be, which is fun if you want to serve in a bowl and top with some fruit.

Give It a Whirl

Depending on your blender, you can add ingredients like apples, pears, cucumbers, and celery stalks whole—seeds and all!—or cored, sliced, chopped, etc.

You don't have to follow these recipes exactly. Experiment and have fun. Swap out water for a nut milk or a banana for an avocado. Out of mango? Use pineapple instead. You can also adjust the sweetness of the recipe by adding more or less stevia or even a dried date or two. Alternatively, adding more greens will cut down on the sweetness. And lastly, smoothies are a perfect way to take your superfoods. Add some soaked chia seeds, hemp seeds, flaxseeds, or maca to any of the recipes for an extra boost. Using fresh or frozen fruit is up to you. Smoothies are always best enjoyed right after you make them, but they'll last in the refrigerator for up to 3 days.

The Alkalizer Smoothie

Yield: 1 quart

2 large stalks celery

1 large handful spinach

1 small lemon, peeled

1 medium pear

2 cups water

In a high-speed blender, blend celery, spinach, lemon, pear, and water until creamy.

Apple Salad Smoothie

Yield: 1 quart

1 large banana

1 large Fuji or other sweet variety apple

1½ cups kale, stems removed

2 cups water

In a high-speed blender, blend banana, Fuji apple, kale, and water until creamy.

Blueberry Blast Smoothie

Yield: 1 quart

1 cup blueberries

½ medium lemon, peeled

4 kale leaves, stems removed

2 cups water

In a high-speed blender, blend blueberries, lemon, kale, and water until creamy.

Chard Love Affair Smoothie

Yield: 1 quart

2 large Fuji apples

5 Swiss chard leaves, stems removed

1 small lemon, peeled

2 cups water

In a high-speed blender, blend Fuji apples, Swiss chard, lemon, and water until creamy.

Coco for Cilantro Smoothie
Yield: 1 quart

1 handful cilantro

4 romaine lettuce leaves

½ medium mango, peeled and pitted

1 large banana

½ TB. coconut oil (optional)

2 cups coconut water

In a high-speed blender, blend cilantro, romaine lettuce, mango, banana, coconut oil (if using), and coconut water until creamy.

Creamy Cherry Smoothie
Yield: 1 quart

1 medium banana

1 medium pear

1 cup frozen cherries

1 heaping TB. chia seeds (soaked for at least 15 minutes in about 3 TB. water)

1 TB. spirulina, or 1 cup kale, stems removed

1 cup fresh almond milk

1 cup water

Stevia (optional)

In a high-speed blender, blend banana, pear, cherries, soaked chia seeds, spirulina, almond milk, water, and stevia (if using) until creamy.

Dandy Dandelion Smoothie
Yield: 1 quart

½ bunch dandelion greens

½ medium cucumber, peeled if not organic, and chopped

½ small lemon, peeled

1 medium pear

2 large stalks celery

2 cups water

In a high-speed blender, blend dandelion greens, cucumber, lemon, pear, celery, and water until creamy.

Green Goddess Smoothie
Yield: 1 quart

1 medium banana

1 medium pear

½ cup pineapple

5 romaine lettuce leaves

1 handful cilantro

Juice of ½ lime

1 TB. coconut oil (optional)

2 cups water

In a high-speed blender, blend banana, pear, pineapple, romaine lettuce, cilantro, lime juice, coconut oil (if using), and water until creamy.

Green Mango Smoothie
Yield: 1 quart

2 large mangoes (frozen, about 2 cups fruit)

1½ cups parsley

1 cup romaine lettuce

2 cups water

In a high-speed blender, blend mangoes, parsley, romaine lettuce, and water until creamy.

Hearty Smoothie Love
Yield: 1 quart

1 cup blueberries

1 heaping handful spinach

¼ avocado

1 large banana

1 TB. almond butter

2 cups water or coconut water

In a high-speed blender, blend blueberries, spinach, avocado, banana, almond butter, and water until creamy.

Hemptastic Smoothie
Yield: 1 quart

2 cups spinach

1 large banana

¾ cup pineapple

1 large stalk celery

⅓ cup hemp seeds

½ cup coconut water

1½ cups water

In a high-speed blender, blend spinach, banana, pineapple, celery, hemp seeds, coconut water, and water until creamy.

Lucky Banana Smoothie
Yield: 1 quart

3 medium frozen ripe bananas

5 romaine lettuce leaves

2 cups fresh almond milk

1 heaping TB. chia seeds (soaked for at least 15 minutes in about 3 TB. water)

In a high-speed blender, blend bananas, romaine lettuce, almond milk, and soaked chia seeds until creamy.

Morning Glory Smoothie
Yield: 1 quart

1 large frozen banana
1 cup peach
1 cup kale leaves, stems removed
1 date, pitted
2 cups almond milk

In a high-speed blender, blend banana, peach, kale, date, and almond milk until creamy.

Passion Parsley Smoothie
Yield: 1 quart

½ bunch parsley
1 cup frozen peaches
1 in. piece fresh ginger, peeled
4 large leaves romaine lettuce
2 cups water
Stevia (optional)

In a high-speed blender, blend parsley, peaches, ginger, romaine lettuce, water, and stevia (if using) until creamy.

Pear Party Smoothie
Yield: 1 quart

1 large pear
1 medium banana
¼ small avocado
1 handful spinach
1 handful romaine lettuce leaves
½ TB. ground cinnamon
2 cups water
Stevia (optional)

In a high-speed blender, blend pear, banana, avocado, spinach, romaine lettuce, cinnamon, water, and stevia (if using) until creamy.

Pink 'n' Green Smoothie
Yield: 1 quart

2 small bananas
3 large stalks celery
1 cup raspberries
2 cups water

In a high-speed blender, blend bananas, celery, raspberries, and water until creamy.

Raspberry Creamsicle Smoothie
Yield: 1 quart

1 cup raspberries

1 large banana

2 cups spinach

1 heaping TB. chia seeds (soaked for at least 15 minutes in about 3 TB. water)

2 cups water

In a high-speed blender, blend raspberries, banana, spinach, soaked chia seeds, and water until creamy.

Southern Bliss Smoothie
Yield: 1 quart

1 small banana

½ large mango, peeled and chopped

1 cup pineapple

4 to 6 collard green leaves, stems removed

2 TB. ground flaxseeds

2 cups water

In a high-speed blender, blend banana, mango, pineapple, collard greens, flaxseeds, and water until creamy.

Spicy Peach Smoothie
Yield: 1 quart

1 medium banana

1 medium peach

1 small kiwifruit

2 cups arugula

2 TB. ground flaxseeds

2 cups water

In a high-speed blender, blend banana, peach, kiwifruit, arugula, flaxseeds, and water until creamy.

Super Green Smoothie
Yield: 1 quart

½ medium lemon, peeled

5 (½-in.-thick) slices cucumber

1 cup spinach

½ cup parsley

2 cups water

In a high-speed blender, blend lemon, cucumbers, spinach, parsley, and water until creamy.

Superfood Smoothie
Yield: 1 quart

1 large banana
1 cup blueberries
1 cup kale
⅓ cup hemp seeds
1 TB. almond butter
1 TB. maca powder

1 TB. goji berries (soaked for at least 15 minutes in about ¼ cup water)
2 cups coconut water

In a high-speed blender, blend banana, blueberries, kale, hemp seeds, almond butter, maca powder, goji berries, and coconut water until creamy.

Swiss Cinnamon Smoothie
Yield: 1 quart

1 cup blueberries
1 medium banana
2 Swiss chard leaves, stalks removed
1 tsp. ground cinnamon
1 TB. hemp seeds
2 cups water

In a high-speed blender, blend blueberries, banana, Swiss chard, cinnamon, hemp seeds, and water until creamy.

Tropical Sensation Smoothie
Yield: 1 quart

1 medium banana
1 cup pineapple
1 handful parsley
1 cup spinach
2 cups water

In a high-speed blender, blend banana, pineapple, parsley, spinach, and water until creamy.

Juices

What's the difference between a freshly made juice and a smoothie? We get that question quite often.

When you make a juice, you use a machine—a juicer—to remove the fiber from the vegetable or fruit. What's left is pure juice goodness, especially when you focus on dark green leafy vegetables. Drinking just the juice requires even less work for your body to absorb and assimilate all the antioxidants, vitamins, minerals, and enzymes than if you were to drink the whole blended vegetable or fruit. This means faster detoxification (the antioxidants bind to toxins), more elimination (bye-bye toxins and old waste matter), alkalization, a healthy glow, decreased inflammation, and more energy!

And a juice quite often contains a lot of fresh food (like a head of kale or celery and big bunch of carrots—that's a lot of food!) so they're quite filling and satisfying.

Don't have a juicer? No problem! Fortunately, juice bars are popping up all over, so hopefully there's one near you. For about the price it would cost you to make it at home (not including the purchase of the juicer), you can order off the menu or bring your book along and ask them to make one of these recipes.

ABC Juice

Yield: 2 cups

2 medium Fuji or other sweet apples

1 medium beet

1 head celery

In a juicer, combine Fuji apples (seeds and all), beet, and celery. Pour into a large glass, and enjoy.

The Elixir

Yield: 2 cups

2 medium cucumbers

2 stalks celery

½ head kale

1 large Granny Smith apple

In a juicer, combine cucumbers, celery, kale, and Granny Smith apple. Pour into a large glass, and enjoy.

The Green Lemon Juice

Yield: 2 cups

½ head romaine lettuce

4 stalks kale

1 large cucumber

1 medium Granny Smith apple

1 lemon, peeled

1 (1-in.) piece fresh ginger, peeled

In a juicer, combine romaine lettuce, kale, cucumber, Granny Smith apple, lemon, and ginger. Pour into a large glass, and enjoy.

Variation: For a sweeter juice, use 2 apples.

Ode to David Wolfe Juice

Yield: 2 cups

1 large cucumber

2 medium apples, any variety

1 large beet

1 large stalk celery

1 medium lemon, peeled

1 large carrot

In a juicer, combine cucumber, apples, beet, celery, lemon, and carrot. Pour into a large glass, and enjoy.

Sweet Spinach Juice

Yield: 2 cups

1 bunch spinach

2 medium Fuji apples

½ medium lemon, peeled

In a juicer, combine spinach, Fuji apples, and lemon. Pour into a large glass, and enjoy.

Herbal Infusions

Herbal infusions can help you take your health to an entirely new level. They're an easy and inexpensive way to load up on minerals and vitamins that will tone, nourish, and detoxify your body.

The first step in successful herbal infusion making is to find high-quality herbs. Check your local health food store for herbs sold in bulk. Plenty of online resources are also available. One of our favorites is Frontier Co-op (frontiercoop.com).

Making herbal infusions isn't difficult, and you have a few different ways you can make them.

Option 1: Fill a quart-size mason jar with loose herbs. Pour hot water over the herbs, and let them steep for at least 10 minutes. Using a handheld strainer, strain your "tea" into your favorite mug (or another mason jar). Compost or discard the herbs.

In Hot Water

When heating water for herbal infusions, we've found it's good to boil your water and then let it cool for a few minutes so it doesn't scorch the herbs.

Option 2: If you have a French press that's been collecting dust since your cleanse started, pull it out, give it a rinse, and put your loose herbs at the bottom. Fill with hot water, and steep for at least 10 minutes. Press, pour, and enjoy!

Option 3: Brew your herbal infusions in your favorite teapot. You can add the herbs to a tea strainer, but be sure the basket is large enough to let the herbs breathe. Then, just follow the preceding instructions.

It's best to drink infusions right after you brew them, but they will keep in the refrigerator for up to 3 days if necessary.

The art of herbal infusions can, and has, filled books by itself. The recipes in this chapter were contributed by renowned herbalist Brigitte Mars, nutritional consultant; instructor at the Omega Institute and Naropa University; and author of many books, including *Beauty by Nature, The Sexual Herbal, Healing Herbal Teas, The Desktop Guide to Herbal Medicine, The Country Almanac of Home Remedies,* and *Rawsome!* For more information, please visit her website at brigittemars.com.

Addiction-Free Tea

Yield: 1 quart

Cinnamon bark

Lemon balm herb

Oatstraw

Spearmint leaf

Choose any 3 ingredients, and use 1 heaping teaspoon of each to make your herbal infusion. Add hot water, and steep for 10 minutes. Pour into your favorite teacup, and enjoy.

Cut the Cravings

The herbs used in this tea help reduce your cravings for harmful substances.

Fasting Tea

Yield: 1 quart

Dandelion root

Fennel seed

Nettle leaf

Peppermint leaf

Red clover blossoms

Choose any 3 ingredients, and use 1 heaping teaspoon of each to make your herbal infusion. Add hot water, and steep for 10 minutes. Pour into your favorite teacup, and enjoy.

Cleanse and Curb

This tea helps cleanse your body and curb your appetite. Be sure to sip it slowly!

Laxative Tea

Yield: 1 quart

Burdock root
Dandelion root
Fennel seed
Licorice root
Raisins

Choose any 3 ingredients, and use 1 heaping teaspoon of each to make your herbal infusion. Add hot water, and steep for 10 minutes. Pour into your favorite teacup, and enjoy.

Clean and Clear

Backed up? This tea will cleanse and nourish your colon.

Spring Cleansing Tea

Yield: 1 quart

1 heaping tsp. dried nettle leaves

1 heaping tsp. dried spearmint leaves

1 heaping tsp. dried violet leaves and flowers

1 tsp. dried unsprayed rose petals, white heels removed

½ tsp. slightly crushed anise seed

In a mason jar, French press, or teapot, combine nettle leaves, spearmint leaves, violet leaves and flowers, rose petals, and anise seed. Add hot water, and steep for 10 minutes. Remove herbs and enjoy, sipping slowly.

Weight Loss Tea

Yield: 1 quart

Burdock root
Dandelion leaf
Fennel seed
Nettle leaf
Raspberry leaf
Yerba mate (optional)

Choose any 3 ingredients, and use 1 heaping teaspoon of each to make your herbal infusion. Add hot water, and steep for 10 minutes. Pour into your favorite teacup, and enjoy.

Stimulating Yerba Mate

Yerba mate isn't suggested during the cleanse because it's a stimulant. But it's great to enjoy when you're not cleansing!

Other Beverages

In this chapter, we give you a few different beverages to enjoy. We also show you ways you can make your own milk replacements and some other special treats to create even more diversity during your cleanse.

These are easier to make than you might expect, and once you experiment a little, there's a good chance you'll start getting creative on your own. Any nut can be made into a milk, so have fun—and bottoms up!

Cleansing Kiwi-Tini
Yield: 1 quart

2 cups seeded and chopped
   watermelon

2 medium kiwis, peeled

1 pitted date

1 cup ice cubes

1 kiwi slice or lime wedge

In a high-speed blender, blend watermelon, kiwis, date, and ice on high until smooth. Pour into a martini glass, and garnish with kiwi slice.

Wonderful Watermelon

Great for inflammation and dehydration, watermelon is high in antioxidants like vitamins A and C. This is a refreshing drink for a hot summer day and perfect for social gatherings.

Homemade Almond Milk

Yield: 4 cups

1 cup raw almonds, soaked in water overnight

4 cups filtered water

Pinch sea salt

2 or 3 dates, pitted, or ¼ cup raw honey

Dash vanilla or almond extract (optional)

In a high-speed blender, blend soaked almonds and filtered water on high for about 2 minutes. Strain almond milk through a nut milk bag. Rinse the blender cup, and pour in almond milk. Add sea salt, dates, and vanilla extract (if using), and blend to combine. Taste for sweetness. Store in a large glass jar in the refrigerator for up to 5 days.

Nutty for Nut Milk

Looking for a great nut milk bag? Find one at our website, consciouscleanse.com.

Homemade Hemp Milk

Yield: 3 cups

3 cups filtered water

1 cup hemp seeds, shelled

1 tsp. vanilla extract (optional)

5 to 10 drops stevia

Pinch sea salt

In a high-speed blender, blend filtered water, hemp seeds, vanilla extract (if using), stevia, and sea salt until smooth and creamy. Store in the refrigerator for up to 5 days.

The Easiest Nut Milk Ever

We love this recipe because it's all one step, with no soaking, no nut bag, and no mess. If you're out of hemp seeds, ½ cup almond butter works just as well as the hemp seeds.

Mango Bubble Drink
Yield: 1 quart

2 cups filtered water

¼ cup chia seeds

1 cup frozen mango

1 banana, peeled and frozen

1 cup almond milk, or your nut
  milk of choice

5 to 7 drops stevia

¼ cup fresh blueberries

In a medium bowl, whisk together filtered water and chia seeds. Let sit for 5 minutes at room temperature, and whisk again. Let sit for 10 more minutes, and whisk again. Meanwhile, in a high-speed blender, blend mango, banana, almond milk, and stevia until smooth. In the bottom of a large glass, place ½ cup chia gel and blueberries. Pour mango and almond milk mixture on top. Enjoy with a wide-mouth straw. Refrigerate any leftover chia gel in a glass container with a tight-fitting lid for up to 2 weeks.

Spiced Chai Tea
Yield: 1 quart

½ tsp. ground cloves

¼ tsp. ground cinnamon

Pinch nutmeg

4 cups almond milk

1 TB. honey (optional)

In a medium saucepan over low heat, combine cloves, cinnamon, nutmeg, and almond milk until warm. Be careful not to let mixture come to a boil to maintain enzymes and integrity of almond milk. Using a handheld strainer, pour tea into a quart jar, discard spices, and add honey (if using).

Variation: This tea is best when made with homemade almond milk, but feel free to substitute commercial almond milk or hemp seed milk instead. You can also adjust the spices to taste.

Warm and Spicy

This tea is a great healthy treat when it's cold outside.

Spicy Lemon Elixir

Yield: 1 quart

4 cups filtered water

Juice of 1 lemon

Pinch cayenne

$\frac{1}{2}$ tsp. local honey, or a few drops
  stevia

In a quart jar, combine filtered
water, lemon juice, cayenne, and
honey. Drink slowly.

Excellent Elixir

This is a variation on the classic "Master Cleanse" drink. It's
an excellent beverage to have first thing in the morning before
breakfast to aid in detoxification. The lemon stimulates bile
release and has a cleansing effect on the digestive tract. The
cayenne stimulates circulation both in the digestive tract and
throughout the body. The honey provides a rapidly absorbed
source of energy. It's best to drink it on an empty stomach.

Breakfasts

In this chapter, we give you a few alternatives or supplements to your green smoothie breakfast regimen. Remember, there's no law against having a salad for breakfast or a brown rice and veggie stir-fry. Just because it's morning doesn't mean you can't feed yourself whatever your body is asking for!

Better-Than-Yogurt Chia Pudding
Yield: 2 cups

1½ cups Homemade Almond Milk
½ cup chia seeds
1½ TB. agave nectar
½ tsp. vanilla extract
⅛ tsp. ground cinnamon
Pinch sea salt

In a medium bowl, combine Homemade Almond Milk, chia seeds, agave nectar, vanilla extract, cinnamon, and sea salt. Let sit and soak at room temperature for 20 minutes, or cover and refrigerate overnight for a yummy breakfast the next day.

Variation: If you like, substitute a commercial unsweetened nut milk or hemp seed milk for the Homemade Almond Milk.

Fresh Fruit and Sweet Banana-Cado
Yield: 8 cups

½ pineapple, peeled, cored, and cubed
1 apple, sliced
½ bunch red seedless grapes
1 pt. fresh raspberries
Sweet Banana-Cado Dip

In a bowl, combine pineapple, apple, red grapes, and raspberries. Serve with a small bowl of Sweet Banana-Cado Dip.

Delightful Dipping

This recipe is a good one for wowing guests at any type of party or brunch. You'll love the look on your guests' faces when you tell them this dish is cleanse friendly.

Raw Apple Walnut Porridge

Yield: 3 cups

1 large Fuji apple, cored and
   chopped roughly
1 cup fresh raspberries
2½ cups Homemade Hemp Milk
½ cup raw walnuts, shelled
½ tsp. vanilla extract
Pinch sea salt
1 tsp. ground cinnamon

In a high-speed blender or a food processor fitted with an S blade, pulse Fuji apple, raspberries, Homemade Hemp Milk, raw walnuts, vanilla extract, and sea salt to desired consistency (between smooth and chunky). Pour into bowls, top with a few extra raspberries and walnuts, and finish with a sprinkle of cinnamon.

Variation: You could also substitute Homemade Almond Milk or commercial unsweetened coconut milk for the Homemade Hemp Milk. Or swap out the raspberries with blackberries or blueberries. You can also replace the walnuts with pecans, raw macadamia nuts, or even almond butter in a pinch.

Easy In, Easy Out

This recipe might not seem ideal when using easy in, easy out food combing principles, but it works because the nuts and fruit are blended and somewhat "predigested" for you. If you have any gas or stomach problems, avoid this combination.

Raw Buckwheat Breakfast Porridge

Yield: 4 cups

2 cups raw buckwheat groats,
   thoroughly rinsed under cold
   water
4 cups filtered water
¼ cup raw honey, or 2 soft dates,
   pitted
1¼ cups unsweetened almond milk
1 tsp. vanilla extract
½ tsp. ground cinnamon
Pinch sea salt

In a medium bowl, soak raw buckwheat groats in filtered water for at least 1 hour or overnight. In a food processor fitted with an S blade or a high-speed blender, combine drained buckwheat groats, raw honey, almond milk, vanilla extract, cinnamon, and sea salt. Transfer to bowls, top with extra cinnamon or almond milk for a thinner consistency, and serve.

In the Raw

Be sure to buy *raw* buckwheat groats. These are different from toasted buckwheat.

Simple Breakfast Porridge
Yield: 2 cups

2 cups cooked brown rice
¼ cup filtered water
1 tsp. maple syrup
1 tsp. ground cinnamon
Pinch sea salt

In a medium saucepan over medium-low heat, combine cooked brown rice, filtered water, maple syrup, cinnamon, and sea salt. Bring to a boil, reduce heat to low, and simmer, stirring occasionally, for about 10 minutes. Remove from heat, and serve.

Viva la Leftovers!

This is a great and easy recipe to use up your leftover brown rice from the night before.

Salads

One of the staples of the Conscious Cleanse is salads. We love a huge salad, but we know some people can get tired of bowls full of green. That won't be the case with the recipes in this chapter!

When getting creative and trying something new, salad-wise—which we encourage you to do!—remember these tips:

- Start with a large, colorful bowl you love.
- Use the ingredients you have in the fridge.
- Make a great dressing.
- Don't forget the sprouts!
- Top with some seeds, nuts, or protein of choice.

A Note on Dressing Your Salad

We believe in making salads ahead of time to cut down on preparation time—it's often a good idea to make more than you'll eat so your next meal is ready and waiting for you. Because of that, it's also a good idea to wait to dress each individual salad you make when you're ready to eat. We suggest using 1 or 2 tablespoons of dressing per individual salad serving.

Remember, for easy in, easy out food combinations, be mindful of your protein selection. If you're adding animal protein, skip the nuts and beans. If you're going to eat nuts and seeds, eat only nuts and seeds. If you want to top a salad with chickpeas, skip the walnuts and chicken.

The Conscious Cleanse "Super Big Easy Salad"
Yield: 1 salad

2 or 3 large fistfuls spinach, arugula, romaine, or a combination

1 cup radishes, cucumbers, carrots, sprouts, fresh herbs, or your favorite mixed vegetables

1 or 2 TB. hemp seeds, ground flaxseeds, walnuts, cashews, or your favorite seeds or nuts

1 or 2 TB. freshly squeezed lemon juice

1 or 2 TB. hemp seed or flaxseed oil

Sea salt

Freshly ground black pepper

In a large bowl, combine spinach, mixed vegetables, and hemp seeds. In a small bowl, combine lemon juice, hemp seed oil, sea salt, and black pepper. Toss salad with dressing and serve.

Whatever's-in-the-Fridge Salad

This is a basic catch-all salad, so top it as you see fit or based on what's in your refrigerator. For extra decadence, try it with ½ an avocado.

Blue Arugula Salad
Yield: 2 salads

3 cups arugula

1 cup alfalfa or your favorite sprouts

¼ cup sunflower seeds

¼ cup Blueberry Bliss Dressing

In a large bowl, combine arugula, alfalfa sprouts, and sunflower seeds. Serve with Blueberry Bliss Dressing.

Caesar Salad
Yield: 2 salads

1 head romaine lettuce, chopped

1 cup celery, chopped

½ cup fennel, chopped

¼ cup Garlic Caesar Dressing

In a large bowl, combine romaine lettuce, celery, and fennel. Toss with Garlic Caesar Dressing, and serve.

Variation: Toss in your favorite protein. We like ½ cup chickpeas, 4 ounces sliced chicken, ½ can sardines, or ¼ cup macadamia nuts with this salad. Another nice topper is ¼ avocado, sliced.

Chopped Italian Salad

Yield: 2 salads

1 head romaine lettuce, chopped
½ cucumber, chopped
½ zucchini, julienned
¼ cup red onion, thinly sliced
½ cup kalamata olives
½ cup chickpeas (optional)
¼ cup Italian Herb Dressing
¼ cup fresh basil, shredded

In a large bowl, top romaine lettuce with cucumber, zucchini, red onion, kalamata olives, and chickpeas (if using). Toss with Italian Herb Dressing, top with fresh basil, and serve.

Golden Beet Salad

Yield: 2 salads

8 golden beets, peeled, and chopped into bite-size pieces
4 TB. olive oil plus more for drizzling
¾ cup walnuts
½ cup raspberry or red wine vinegar
1 TB. maple syrup or agave nectar
¼ cup chickpeas
Sea salt
Freshly ground black pepper
1 shallot, thinly sliced
¼ cup fresh cilantro or parsley, finely chopped
2 cups arugula, chopped
1 cup sunflower sprouts

Preheat the oven to 350°F. Place golden beets in a baking dish, and drizzle with a little olive oil. Cover with aluminum foil, and bake for about 25 minutes or until soft. Meanwhile, in a high-speed blender, blend ½ cup walnuts, remaining 4 tablespoons olive oil, raspberry vinegar, maple syrup, and chickpeas. Remove beets from the oven, and toss with sea salt and black pepper. Place cooked golden beets, shallot, and cilantro in a large salad bowl, and toss with salad dressing. Marinate in the refrigerator for at least 1 hour or up to 3 days. Serve beets over arugula, and garnish with sunflower sprouts and remaining ¼ cup walnuts.

Kale Avocado Salad with a Kick

Yield: 2 salads

1 bunch curly kale, chopped and destemmed

1 avocado, sliced

1 TB. freshly squeezed lemon juice

3 TB. olive oil

2 pinches sea salt

Dash cayenne

In a large bowl, place kale and avocado. In a small bowl, combine lemon juice, olive oil, sea salt, and cayenne. Pour dressing over kale and avocado, massage kale thoroughly with your hands until it becomes soft, and serve.

Variation: This salad is terrific as is, or even better with a variety of hemp seeds, sprouts, sliced cucumber, and/or shredded carrots added in.

Kale Seaweed Salad

Yield: 2 salads

½ cup arame sea vegetables

1 head lacinato (dinosaur) kale, destemmed and chopped

3 TB. sesame oil

¼ cup brown rice vinegar

1 TB. minced garlic

1 TB. peeled and minced fresh ginger

½ TB. honey

3 large carrots, shredded

1 TB. seaweed gomasio

Rinse arame sea vegetables, place in a bowl, cover with water, and let soak for at least 5 to 10 minutes. Meanwhile, in a large salad bowl, combine lacinato kale and 1 tablespoon sesame oil. Massage kale thoroughly using your hands until it begins to wilt and soften. In a jar, combine remaining 2 tablespoons sesame oil, brown rice vinegar, garlic, ginger, and honey, and shake vigorously. Drain arame, and add to kale. Toss with dressing, carrots, and seaweed gomasio, and serve immediately or chill.

Variation: If you're craving something warm, you can always lightly sauté your oil, garlic, and ginger. Then, add the plain kale, and sauté for a few minutes. Toss in the arame, carrots, and dressing, and warm slightly.

Rainbow Salad
Yield: 2 salads

4 cups arugula, spinach, mixed baby greens, or your favorite greens

½ cup zucchini, shredded

½ cup red cabbage, shredded

½ cup carrots, shredded

½ cup alfalfa, broccoli, sunflower, or your favorite sprouts

¼ cup Balsamic Vinaigrette

Place arugula in the center of a plate, and arrange piles of zucchini, red cabbage, carrots, and alfalfa sprouts around it. Drizzle with Balsamic Vinaigrette, and serve.

Variation: This salad works with any veggies you've got in the fridge. Just shred them and place them around a bed of greens. You could add a side of hummus or kalamata olive tapenade around the edge of plate as well.

Quick and Easy

This is a great salad to make for yourself when you're short on time! You can use a traditional cheese grater or your food processor to shred the veggies.

Salad Niçoise

Yield: 2 salads

½ cup water

½ lb. green beans, ends trimmed

1 bunch asparagus, ends trimmed

1½ TB. apple cider vinegar

½ TB. Dijon mustard

½ cup olive oil

1 clove garlic, minced

1 shallot, finely chopped

1 TB. fresh rosemary, finely chopped

1 TB. fresh tarragon, finely chopped

Pinch sea salt

Freshly ground black pepper

5 cups mixed baby greens

2 lemon wedges

½ cup niçoise, kalamata, or your favorite variety olives

In a sauté pan over medium-high heat, combine water, green beans, and asparagus. Cover and steam for about 5 minutes or until soft. When finished, drain off water (or drink it!) and set aside green beans and asparagus. In a small bowl, whisk together apple cider vinegar and Dijon mustard until well combined. Slowly whisk in olive oil. Stir in garlic, shallot, rosemary, and tarragon. Add sea salt and black pepper. In a large salad bowl, toss mixed baby greens with about ⅓ cup salad dressing. In another medium bowl, toss asparagus and green beans with drizzle of salad dressing. Adjust dressing to taste. To assemble salads, arrange baby greens in the center of a plate, top with several pieces of asparagus, and add a large helping of green beans to the side. Garnish with lemon wedges and a small handful of fresh olives, drizzle a small amount of dressing across the entire plate, and top with another pinch of sea salt (optional) and black pepper.

Variation: You could also serve this salad with 4 to 8 ounces grilled tuna.

Keep It Cool

Chill your plates ahead of time to keep this salad cold and crisp.

The Shredded Salad

Yield: 4 salads

6 carrots, grated
3 stalks celery, sliced or grated
3 parsnips, grated
½ head red cabbage, grated
½ cup Citrus Squeeze Dressing
Sea salt
Freshly ground black pepper

In a large bowl, combine carrots, celery, parsnips, and red cabbage. Toss with Citrus Squeeze Dressing, season with sea salt and black pepper, and serve. Or store in a glass storage container in the refrigerator for up to 1 week.

Variation: This salad is great alone or with 1 tablespoon hemp seeds added for protein, ¼ cup Bubbie's sauerkraut for better digestion, or an optional ¼ cup avocado for some healthy and filling fats.

Salads Made Easy

This recipe gives you a week's worth of delicious salads. No chopping, peeling, slicing, or dicing at each mealtime. Just grab your greens, and add The Shredded Salad as a topper to your favorite bed of greens (like The Conscious Cleanse "Super Big Easy Salad"). Drizzle some of your favorite salad dressing, and you're on your way.

Wakame Cucumber Salad

Yield: 6 side salads

1 (2- or 3-oz.) bag wakame sea vegetables
½ cucumber, halved and thinly sliced
2 TB. sesame oil
3 TB. brown rice vinegar
1 TB. peeled and grated fresh ginger
¼ cup sesame seeds

Soak wakame sea vegetables in water for 5 minutes. Drain, place wakame in a bowl, and add cucumber. In a small bowl, combine sesame oil, brown rice vinegar, and ginger. Pour dressing over wakame and cucumbers, and toss to coat. Sprinkle sesame seeds over top of salad. Chill for 20 minutes, and serve cold.

Variation: This salad also works well garnished with ½ cup shredded carrots.

Salad Dressings

A scrumptious salad dressing makes all the difference in keeping things interesting and satisfying in the salad world. As with anything, we tend to settle into our favorites, and eventually even those start to get old. Trust us: if you find yourself tired or bored with eating salads every day, a new dressing can rekindle your love of greens. Some of the dressings in this chapter are so full of flavor, we actually use them as a dip for veggie sticks. As always, allow yourself to get creative. Add more or less pepper, cayenne, or garlic. And don't be shy with the sea salt. It helps bring out the flavors.

The amount of salad dressing you use is a matter of personal taste, so a word to the wise: drizzle slowly and see what works for you. We generally suggest about 1 or 2 tablespoons per salad. These recipes typically yield 1 or 2 cups dressing, so one batch gives you dressing for a week.

Balsamic Vinaigrette

Yield: 1 cup

¾ cup olive oil

¼ cup balsamic vinegar

½ clove garlic, minced

1 tsp. Dijon mustard

½ tsp. sea salt

½ tsp. freshly ground black pepper

Dash stevia (optional)

In a small bowl, whisk together olive oil, balsamic vinegar, garlic, Dijon mustard, sea salt, and black pepper. Sweeten with stevia (if using). Refrigerate in a glass container for 1 week.

Blueberry Bliss Dressing

Yield: 1 cup

1 cup frozen or fresh blueberries

2 pitted dates

2 TB. freshly squeezed lime juice

1 TB. freshly squeezed lemon juice

3 TB. balsamic vinegar

3 TB. filtered water

Pinch sea salt

In a high-speed blender, combine blueberries, dates, lime juice, lemon juice, balsamic vinegar, filtered water, and sea salt. Refrigerate in a glass container for 3 or 4 days.

Citrus Squeeze Dressing

Yield: 1 cup

⅓ cup freshly squeezed lemon or lime juice

⅔ cup olive, flaxseed, or hemp seed oil

Sea salt

Dash cayenne

In a medium bowl, whisk together lemon juice, olive oil, sea salt, and cayenne. Store in a glass container for 5 to 7 days.

Variation: For a slightly different approach, squeeze a generous amount of lemon or lime juice over your salad, add a drizzle of olive, flaxseed, or hemp seed oil, and sprinkle with cayenne and your favorite fresh or dried herbs.

Dill Vinaigrette Dressing

Yield: 1½ cups

3 TB. apple cider vinegar

3 TB. fresh dill, or to taste

1 cup filtered water

¼ cup olive oil

5 drops stevia

In a high-speed blender, blend apple cider vinegar, dill, filtered water, olive oil, and stevia until creamy. Refrigerate in a glass container for up to 7 days.

East-Meets-West Dressing

Yield: 2 cups

¼ cup freshly squeezed lime juice

1 clove garlic

⅓ cup fresh cilantro

¼ cup chickpeas

1 tsp. honey (optional)

¼ cup olive oil

Sea salt

Freshly ground black pepper

In a high-speed blender, combine lime juice, garlic, cilantro, chickpeas, and honey (if using). With the blender running, gradually drizzle in olive oil. Season with sea salt and black pepper. Refrigerate in a glass container for up to 3 days.

Garlic Caesar Dressing

Yield: 1 cup

1 cup cashews, soaked in water for 2 hours

2 cloves garlic, chopped

¼ tsp. sea salt

2 TB. freshly squeezed lemon juice

3 soft dates, pitted

¾ cups water

2 large stalks celery, chopped

Freshly ground black pepper

In high-speed blender, combine cashews, garlic, sea salt, lemon juice, dates, water, celery, and black pepper. Refrigerate in a glass container for 2 or 3 days.

Soak to Soften

If your dates are on the hard side, soak them in water for 10 minutes before draining and adding to the dressing.

Italian Herb Dressing

Yield: 1½ cups

1 TB. honey

1 TB. Dijon mustard

2 TB. freshly squeezed lemon juice

1 cup olive oil

1 clove garlic, minced

⅛ tsp. dried parsley

⅛ tsp. dried oregano

⅛ tsp. dried basil

Pinch sea salt

½ tsp. freshly ground black pepper

In a glass jar with a lid, stir together honey and Dijon mustard with a spoon until well combined. Add lemon juice, olive oil, garlic, parsley, oregano, basil, sea salt, and black pepper; screw on lid; and shake vigorously. Refrigerate for up to 5 days.

Fantastic Fresh Herbs

If you have an herb garden and can substitute fresh herbs for dried, by all means do so! It may work best to use your blender to ensure the herbs are well combined with the rest of the ingredients. You'll usually use about three times the quantity of fresh as you would dried herbs.

Sunny Sunflower Dressing

Yield: 3 cups

2 carrots, peeled

1 cup sunflower seeds, soaked in water for 2 hours

1½ cups water

2 tsp. minced garlic, or 1 tsp. garlic granules

1 tsp. sea salt

⅛ to ¼ tsp. cayenne

¾ cup olive oil

In a high-speed blender, blend carrots, sunflower seeds, water, garlic, sea salt, and cayenne on the highest setting until smooth. (When it comes to cayenne, a little goes a long way, so start with ⅛ teaspoon and add more to taste.) Turn blender to medium setting, slowly add olive oil, and blend until creamy and smooth. Refrigerate in a glass jar for 3 to 7 days. Fresh garlic spoils faster than garlic granules, so if you use fresh garlic, refrigerate dressing for up to 3 days.

Soups

Soups play an important role in the cleansing process. They make great evening meals because they tend to be blended, warm, and nourishing, which supports easy digestion. Soups are light, but they're also filling and satisfying.

You may wonder how you'll possibly enjoy your soup without your usual side of bread. The answer? Raw crackers! They're excellent soup companions, highly nutritious, and cleanse friendly.

Bieler's Broth

Yield: 2 large bowls

2 medium zucchini, chopped
3 stalks celery, chopped
1 large handful frozen or fresh green beans
1 large handful spinach (optional)
2 cups water
1 handful fresh parsley

In a large stockpot over medium-high heat, steam zucchini, celery, and green beans in water for about 10 minutes or until they're very soft. Add spinach (if using) at the end and steam for only about 2 minutes. Place veggies, remaining steaming water in the stockpot, and uncooked parsley into a blender and blend for 1 or 2 minutes until smooth. Eat this broth fresh from the blender for the best taste.

Variation: You can substitute with more spinach if green beans are unavailable. When you're not fasting, Bieler's Broth makes a rich, wholesome base you can add other ingredients and flavors to. You also can flavor it to your liking by adding oil, sautéed onions, garlic, and other vegetables such as broccoli, additional chopped zucchini and celery, and snow peas. Or flavor with sea salt and black pepper or cayenne.

Chilled Cucumber Dill Soup

Yield: 2 large bowls

1 ripe avocado, pitted

1 large cucumber, peeled if not organic

4 TB. fresh dill, or to taste

Juice of ½ lemon

½ tsp. sea salt

1 or 2 TB. water

In a high-speed blender, mix avocado, cucumber, dill, lemon juice, and sea salt until smooth. Add 1 or 2 tablespoons water as needed to make creamier. Chill soup for at least 20 minutes before serving.

Curried Carrot Soup

Yield: 8 bowls

3 TB. coconut oil

2 tsp. curry powder

8 medium carrots, peeled and sliced thin

4 medium stalks celery, chopped

1 medium yellow onion, coarsely chopped

5 cups vegetable broth

1 TB. freshly squeezed lemon juice

2 tsp. sea salt

Freshly ground black pepper

In a medium saucepan over low heat, cook coconut oil and curry powder, stirring, for 2 minutes. Stir in carrots, celery, and yellow onion; toss to coat; and cook, stirring frequently, for 10 minutes. Stir in vegetable broth, bring to a boil, reduce heat to low, and simmer for 10 minutes or until vegetables are very tender. Allow to sit for 1 minute, and skim grease from top of soup. In a blender, and working in batches of no more than 2 cups, purée soup. Return soup to the pot, and heat through. Season with lemon juice, sea salt, and black pepper, and serve. Refrigerate leftover soup in a glass container for 3 days.

Two Meals in One

For a second meal, pour 1 cup Curried Carrot Soup over 1 or 2 cups of your favorite nongluten grain.

Hearty Vegetable Stew

Yield: 8 bowls

3 TB. coconut oil

1 large yellow onion, diced

4 stalks celery, chopped

4 carrots, chopped

6 parsnips, chopped

2 cloves garlic, minced

2 (14.5-oz.) cans white beans, drained and rinsed

1 bay leaf

2 or 3 qt. vegetable stock

2 cups brussels sprouts, stems removed and cut in ½

2 bunches kale and/or collard greens, stems removed and chopped

1 large sprig rosemary

In a large soup pot over medium heat, heat coconut oil. Add yellow onion and celery, stir, and cook for 2 minutes. Add carrots and parsnips, stir, and cook for 5 minutes. Add garlic, white beans, and bay leaf, and stir for 1 minute. Add vegetable stock until it covers ingredients by 1 inch. Bring to boil. Add brussels sprouts and kale, along with more vegetable stock if necessary, and bring to a boil. Reduce heat to low and simmer for 10 minutes. Remove pot from heat, add rosemary, cover, and let sit for 15 minutes. Remove rosemary and bay leaf, and serve.

Raw Broccoli Soup

Yield: 5 bowls

4 cups Homemade Almond Milk

2 cups broccoli, stems and florets

1 stalk celery

1 avocado, halved and pitted

1 clove garlic, minced

1 TB. olive oil

1½ tsp. sea salt

½ tsp. cumin

¼ tsp. freshly ground black pepper

In a high-speed blender, combine Homemade Almond Milk, broccoli, celery, avocado, garlic, olive oil, sea salt, cumin, and black pepper until creamy. To warm soup more, blend for up to 5 minutes.

Raw Carrot Soup

Yield: 6 bowls

3 cups filtered water

3 medium carrots

1 medium Fuji apple

1 (1- or 2-in.) piece fresh ginger, peeled

1 avocado, halved and pitted

1 large handful fresh cilantro

1 or 2 TB. freshly squeezed lemon juice

1 date, pitted

1 tsp. ground cumin

¼ tsp. sea salt

¼ tsp. freshly ground black pepper

Pinch cayenne

In a high-speed blender, blend filtered water, carrots, Fuji apple, ginger, avocado, cilantro, lemon juice, date, cumin, sea salt, black pepper, and cayenne until creamy. To warm soup more, blend for up to 5 minutes.

Red Chard and White Bean Soup

Yield: 8 bowls

2 TB. olive oil

1 yellow onion, finely chopped

2 medium bunches red chard, leaves, stems, and ribs chopped

2 cloves garlic, minced

4 cups vegetable broth

3 cups cooked or canned cannellini or white kidney beans (drained and rinsed if canned)

1 bay leaf

1 sprig thyme

In a large soup pot over medium-high heat, heat olive oil. Add yellow onion and red chard, ribs and stems only, saving leaves; sprinkle lightly with sea salt; reduce heat to medium; and sauté for about 10 minutes or until vegetables are softened. Add garlic, and cook, stirring frequently, for 1 or 2 more minutes or until garlic is fragrant. Add vegetable broth, and bring to a simmer. Stir in cannellini beans and add remaining red chard leaves along with bay leaf and thyme. Cover and simmer for 5 to 7 minutes or until chard leaves are wilted and tender to bite. Immediately remove bay leaf and thyme, and serve.

Red Lentil Soup

Yield: 8 bowls

2 TB. coconut oil
1 TB. mustard seeds
1 tsp. coriander powder
1 TB. curry powder
1 small white onion, diced
2 cloves garlic, minced
1 TB. minced ginger
3 carrots, diced
3 stalks celery, diced
2 cups uncooked red lentils, rinsed
½ tsp. sea salt
Pinch cayenne
Fresh cilantro

In a large pot over medium heat, heat coconut oil, mustard seeds, coriander powder, and curry powder. Add white onion, garlic, and ginger, and sauté for 1 minute. Add carrots, and sauté for 2 or 3 more minutes. Add celery, and sauté for 2 or 3 minutes. Add red lentils along with water to cover lentils by 4 inches. Simmer for about 30 minutes or until lentils are so tender they break down and become creamy. If soup is too thick, add more water at this point. Season with sea salt, and simmer for 10 more minutes. Garnish with cilantro and cayenne just before serving.

Zesty Watermelon Gazpacho

Yields: 6 bowls

5 cups seedless watermelon, cubed
1 small cucumber, peeled and diced
3 celery stalks, chopped
½ small red onion, diced
¼ cup fresh mint leaves
1 small jalapeño
1 clove garlic
3 TB. freshly squeezed lime juice
1 (1- or 2-in.) piece fresh ginger, peeled
½ tsp. sea salt

Set aside a handful of watermelon, cucumber, celery, red onion, mint leaves, and jalapeño, and dice finely to use as garnish. In a high-speed blender, blend remaining watermelon, cucumber, celery, red onion, garlic, mint leaves, lime juice, ginger, jalapeño, and sea salt until creamy. Transfer to a bowl, cover with plastic wrap, and refrigerate for at least 2 hours. Serve cold with a few tablespoons garnish in each bowl. Season with more fresh mint leaves and sea salt to taste.

Snacks

We love snacks! If you follow the simple rule of eating when you're truly hungry as opposed to snacking out of habit, you'll be well on your way to vibrant health.

The best snacks require little to no preparation at all—banana slices with almond butter, a handful of walnuts, etc. But sometimes you want a little extra something special or a treat that can wow guests. That's just what you'll find in this chapter.

Carrot Chips
Yield: about 40 chips

1 TB. olive oil

¼ tsp. cumin

4 large carrots, peeled, halved, and cut into thin rectangular "chips"

¼ tsp. sea salt

¼ tsp. freshly ground black pepper

Preheat the oven to 250°F. In a small bowl, combine olive oil and cumin. Place carrot chips on a parchment paper–lined baking sheet, drizzle with dressing, and sprinkle with sea salt and black pepper. Toss until thoroughly coated. Bake for about 40 minutes until edges of carrot chips start to turn golden. Served immediately with your favorite dip.

Fruit Salad Supreme
Yield: 3 cups

1 cup peaches, cut into bite-size pieces

½ cup kiwifruit, cut into bite-size pieces

1 cup red or green seedless grapes

1 cup blueberries

1 TB. freshly squeezed lime juice

In a medium bowl, combine peaches, kiwifruit, red grapes, and blueberries. Drizzle with lime juice, and gently toss to coat. Serve immediately, or refrigerate for up to 1 day.

Joy Balls

Yield: 3 dozen balls

1 cup raw sunflower seeds
½ cup tahini
1 cup raw almond butter
1 cup raisins or dates
3 TB. raw honey
¼ cup finely grated, unsweetened coconut flakes (optional)

In a food processor fitted with an S blade, grind sunflower seeds for about 2 minutes or until fairly fine. Add tahini, raw almond butter, raisins, and raw honey, and blend for about 2 minutes or until a thick paste forms. Mixture will be relatively dry. Using your hands, roll small amounts of mixture between your palms to form about 36 (1-inch) balls. Roll balls in coconut flakes (if using). Place in a container with a tight-fitting lid and refrigerate or freeze for a chilly treat. Serve chilled or frozen. These will last up to 2 weeks.

Kale Chips

Yield: 2 cups

1 or 2 TB. olive oil
1 TB. freshly squeezed lime juice
1 bunch lacinato (dinosaur) kale
½ tsp. sea salt

Preheat the oven to 350°F. Line a baking sheet with parchment paper. In a small bowl, combine olive oil and lime juice, and set aside. Rinse and dry lacinato kale thoroughly, using a salad spinner if you have one. (Be sure kale is dry, or you'll have steamed or burned chips.) Remove kale stems, and cut leaves into small pieces. Spread kale on the prepared baking sheet, and drizzle with olive oil–lime juice mixture. Bake for 10 to 12 minutes or until crispy. Stay close to the oven because these can burn very quickly. Remove from the oven and immediately sprinkle with sea salt.

The Perfect Chip?

Here's one chip that there's no shame in snacking on. These are also great to wow your friends with at your next potluck.

Protein-Packed Almond Butter Balls

Yield: about 3 dozen

2 cups medjool dates, pitted

¼ tsp. sea salt

1 tsp. vanilla extract (optional)

¼ cup raw almond butter

¼ cup shredded, unsweetened coconut flakes

¼ cup hemp seeds

In a food processor fitted with an S blade, combine medjool dates, sea salt, vanilla extract (if using), and raw almond butter for 1 to 3 minutes or until a smooth texture is reached. In a small bowl, combine coconut flakes and hemp seeds. Using your hands, roll almond-date mixture into about 36 (1-inch) balls. Roll balls in coconut and hemp seed mixture, and place in a container with a tight-fitting lid. Store in the freezer or refrigerator, and enjoy chilled or frozen.

Raw Trail Mix

Yield: 3 cups

1 cup raw cashews

1 cup raw walnuts

½ cup sunflower seeds

½ cup raisins or goji berries

¼ cup dried apricots, chopped

Pinch sea salt, or to taste

In a medium bowl, combine raw cashews, raw walnuts, sunflower seeds, raisins, and apricots. Season with sea salt. Store in a glass container, or divide into 1-cup portions in small to-go baggies.

Spicy Zucchini Chips

Yield: about 20 chips

1 large zucchini

Pinch cayenne

Pinch sea salt

1 TB. olive oil (optional)

Slice zucchini into bite-size rounds. Sprinkle cayenne and sea salt over one side of each round, and drizzle with olive oil (if using). Serve immediately, or cover and refrigerate for up to 1 day.

Dips and Sauces

Dips and sauces are a great way to add flavor and diversity to your cleanse. When you're feeling as if you can't face another plain old piece of steamed broccoli, you'll be amazed at what happens when you pair it with one of the concoctions from this chapter. Easy to make, and easier to eat, these recipes are also full of nutritious whole ingredients to keep your digestive system humming and your body well fueled.

As always, stay creative and check our website for more great ideas.

Beet Hummus

Yield: 2 cups

3 medium beets, peeled and quartered

2 TB. tahini

¼ cup freshly squeezed lemon juice

1 clove garlic, chopped

¼ cup olive oil plus a drizzle for roasting beets

½ tsp. sea salt

½ tsp. freshly ground black pepper

Preheat oven to 375°F. Place beets in a baking dish, drizzle with olive oil, cover, and bake until soft, about 20 minutes. In a food processor fitted with an S blade, process beets, tahini, lemon juice, garlic, olive oil, sea salt, and black pepper until smooth. Cover and refrigerate for at least 1 hour to allow flavors to develop. Refrigerate for up to 1 week.

Black Bean Hummus

Yield: 2 cups

2 cups cooked black beans

2 cloves garlic, minced

4 TB. olive oil

¼ cup freshly squeezed lemon juice

2 TB. rice wine vinegar

1 tsp. ground cumin

½ tsp. sea salt

Freshly ground black pepper

1 head Bibb lettuce

In a food processor fitted with an S blade, blend black beans, garlic, olive oil, lemon juice, rice wine vinegar, cumin, sea salt, and black pepper for 1 minute or until almost smooth. Cover and chill for 15 minutes before serving with Bibb lettuce. Refrigerate in a glass container for 7 to 10 days.

Tips for Cooking Beans

Cooking beans from scratch isn't as difficult as you might think. It helps to soak the beans. This quickens the cooking time and also makes them easier to digest. To soak, cover 1 part beans with 3 parts water, and let sit overnight. In the morning, drain the beans and cook in fresh water. Also, try cooking the beans with a strip of kombu (sea vegetable) in it. Finally, salt the beans *after* cooking. Don't add salt to boiling water because it will prevent the beans from cooking thoroughly, resulting in tough, undercooked beans.

Chickpea Hummus

Yield: 2 cups

2 cups cooked or canned chickpeas

4 TB. freshly squeezed lemon juice

2 TB. tahini

2 cloves garlic, crushed

4 or 5 TB. olive oil

1 tsp. sea salt

½ jalapeño, seeded (optional)

¼ tsp. cayenne (optional)

¼ cup water

1 TB. fresh parsley, finely chopped (optional)

In a food processor fitted with an S blade, blend chickpeas, lemon juice, tahini, garlic, 3 tablespoons olive oil, sea salt, jalapeño (if using), and cayenne (if using). While blending, add water, and blend for 3 to 5 minutes on low until thoroughly mixed and smooth. Place hummus in a medium shallow bowl, and create a hole in center. Add remaining 1 or 2 tablespoons olive oil in well. Garnish with parsley (if using), and serve. Refrigerate in a glass container for 7 to 10 days.

Kalamata Olive Tapenade

Yield: about 1 cup

1 cup black kalamata olives, pitted

¼ cup olive oil

2 or 3 tsp. freshly squeezed lemon juice

1 tsp. lemon zest

2 cloves garlic, minced

¼ tsp. freshly ground black pepper

In a food processor fitted with an S blade, blend kalamata olives, olive oil, lemon juice, lemon zest, garlic, and black pepper for about 1 minute or until a paste forms. Refrigerate in a glass container for up to 3 weeks.

Sherpa Spinach Dip

Yield: 1 cup

4 cups spinach

1 large avocado, halved and pitted

½ TB. lemon juice

1 small clove garlic, minced

¼ tsp. curry

¼ tsp. cumin

⅛ tsp. fresh peeled and chopped ginger

Dash cayenne

¼ tsp. sea salt, or to taste

In a food processor fitted with an S blade, blend spinach, avocado, lemon juice, garlic, curry, cumin, ginger, cayenne, and sea salt. Serve immediately, with carrot sticks or flaxseed crackers.

Serve Immediately

We recommend you serve this and any other dip containing avocado or banana immediately so these ingredients won't have a chance to turn brown due to oxidation. If you do need to store the dip, cover tightly and scrape off the brown layer before serving.

Simple Basil Pesto

Yield: about 1 cup

1½ cups pine nuts
½ cup fresh basil
1 clove garlic
¼ tsp. sea salt, or to taste
1 tsp. olive oil

In a food processor fitted with an S blade, combine pine nuts, basil, garlic, and sea salt. While mixing, drizzle olive oil into the food processor. Add more oil as needed to blend into a creamy paste. Season with additional sea salt as needed. Refrigerate in a glass container for up to 3 weeks.

Simple Guacamole

Yield: about 1½ cups

2 avocados, halved and pitted
¼ cup freshly squeezed lime juice
2 cloves garlic, finely minced
¼ cup red onion, finely chopped
½ cup fresh cilantro, chopped
1 tsp. jalapeño, seeded and minced (optional)
½ tsp. sea salt
Freshly ground black pepper

Scoop out avocado flesh, and put into a bowl. Using a fork, roughly mash avocados. Add lime juice, garlic, red onion, cilantro, and jalapeño (if using). Season with sea salt and black pepper, and serve immediately to avoid browning.

Sweet Banana-Cado Dip

Yield: 1 cup

1 banana, peeled
1 avocado, halved and pitted
1 clove garlic

In a food processor fitted with an S blade or a blender, blend banana, avocado, and garlic for about 1 minute or until smooth. Eat like pudding with a spoon or serve with flaxseed crackers.

Tahini Dipping Sauce
Yield: 1 cup

½ cup tahini

1 TB. raw honey

¼ cup apple cider vinegar

2 TB. fresh peeled and grated ginger

1 clove garlic, minced

Pinch sea salt

In a small bowl, whisk together tahini, raw honey, apple cider vinegar, ginger, and garlic. Season with sea salt. Refrigerate in a glass container for up to 1 week.

Tropical Mango Salsa
Yield: 4 cups

4 cups diced mango, or 2 cups diced mango and 2 cups peach

3 TB. freshly squeezed lime juice

2 TB. minced ginger

½ cup red onion, chopped

½ jalapeño, seeded and diced

½ tsp. sea salt

¼ cup chopped fresh cilantro

¼ cup small avocado chunks

In a food processor fitted with an S blade, pulse mango, lime juice, ginger, red onion, jalapeño, sea salt, and cilantro. Keep salsa chunky. Garnish with avocado before serving. Refrigerate in a glass container for up to 3 days.

Zucchini Hummus
Yield: about 3 cups

2 medium zucchini, chopped

¾ cup tahini

½ cup freshly squeezed lemon juice

¼ cup olive oil

2 cloves garlic

1½ tsp. sea salt, or to taste

2 TB. cumin

In a food processor fitted with an S blade, blend zucchini, tahini, lemon juice, olive oil, garlic, sea salt, and cumin until smooth and creamy. Refrigerate in a glass container for up to 1 week.

Veggie Dishes

Next to the Green Smoothies chapter, this is by far our favorite chapter. Vegetable-based entrées are "what's for dinner" … and they're also what's for lunch and even breakfast, too!

In the Conscious Cleanse, we encourage participants to think of filling their plate with vegetable dishes for every meal and allowing other foods to be secondary. This small shift in perspective has the power to completely transform your health. Eat your veggies and enjoy!

Cauliflower Mashers with Mushroom Gravy
Yield: 4 to 6 cups

2 cups raw cashews, soaked in water for 2 hours

2⅓ cups water

1 head cauliflower, cored and chopped

¼ medium white onion, quartered

1 tsp. olive oil

2 tsp. sea salt

Pinch freshly ground black pepper

2 cups crimini or portobello mushrooms, chopped

1 clove garlic

¼ tsp. ground dried sage

1 TB. Ume plum vinegar

In a food processor fitted with an S blade, process raw cashews, 1 cup water, cauliflower, white onion, olive oil, 1 teaspoon sea salt, and black pepper until well blended. Remove mixture from the food processor, and place in a bowl. Rinse the food processor, and mix crimini mushrooms, remaining 1 teaspoon sea salt, remaining 1⅓ cups water, garlic, sage, and Ume plum vinegar until smooth. Pour mushroom gravy over cauliflower mashers, and serve cold or slightly warm.

Citus Burst Broccoli

Yield: 3 cups

1 head broccoli (including crowns and stems), chopped

Juice of ½ lemon

½ TB. olive oil

Pinch sea salt

½ avocado, pitted and chopped

Dash seaweed gomasio

Add a steamer basket to a large pot and fill with 1 inch water. Set over medium-high heat, cover, and bring water to a boil. Add broccoli stem pieces, cover, and steam for 2 minutes. Add broccoli crown pieces, cover, and steam for 5 minutes. Meanwhile, in a medium bowl, combine lemon juice, olive oil, and sea salt. Add warm broccoli to the bowl, add avocado, and gently toss. Sprinkle with seaweed gomasio before serving.

Colorful Collard Wraps

Yield: 6 wraps

3 large collard leaves, stems removed, and cut in ½

6 TB. Zucchini Hummus

2 carrots, shredded

1 cup purple cabbage, shredded

1 handful your favorite sprouts

½ avocado, pitted and sliced

¼ cup raw hemp seeds

Wash and dry collard leaf halves. Lay them out flat, and spread 1 tablespoon Zucchini Hummus on one end of each. Layer on shredded carrots, purple cabbage, sprouts, and avocado slices. Sprinkle with raw hemp seeds. Roll, and enjoy.

Variation: This is a great recipe to make with The Shredded Salad, if you have some in the fridge and ready to go.

Fast and Easy Lentils
Yield: 2 cups

1 cup uncooked green or brown lentils

3 cups water

1 TB. coconut oil

½ cup chopped white onion

2 cloves garlic, minced

1 cup zucchini, diced

½ cup spinach, chopped

2 TB. balsamic vinegar

½ tsp. sea salt, or to taste

½ tsp. freshly ground black pepper

Rinse green lentils under cold water and drain. Place in a medium saucepan, pour in water, and set over medium-high heat. Bring to a boil, reduce heat to medium-low, and cook for about 45 minutes or until tender. Meanwhile, in a sauté pan over medium-low heat, heat coconut oil. Add white onion and garlic, and sauté for about 3 minutes or until onions become translucent. Add zucchini, and cook for 5 minutes. Add spinach, and sauté for 2 or 3 minutes or until spinach is slightly wilted. Add cooked lentils, balsamic vinegar, sea salt, and black pepper, and mix well. Serve warm.

Marinated Greens
Yield: 5 cups

2 cups kale

2 cups Swiss chard

2 cups dandelion greens

⅓ cup olive oil

2 TB. Ume plum vinegar

½ cup water

Pinch cayenne (optional)

Wash, dry, and cut kale, Swiss chard, and dandelion greens into bite-size pieces. Set aside. In a high-speed blender fitted with an S blade, blend together olive oil, Ume plum vinegar, water, and cayenne (if using) until mixed well. Pour marinade over greens, and mix well with your hands, massaging greens until they begin to wilt a bit. Cover and let sit at room temperature or in the refrigerator for at least 1 hour before serving.

Marinated Portobello Mushrooms

Yield: 3 mushrooms

¼ cup balsamic vinegar

3 TB. olive oil

3 TB. maple syrup

½ shallot, peeled and diced

Juice of ½ lemon

Pinch sea salt

Pinch freshly ground black pepper

3 portobello mushrooms, stems removed and chopped into 1-in. cubes

In a large bowl, combine balsamic vinegar, olive oil, maple syrup, shallot, lemon juice, sea salt, and black pepper. Add portobello mushrooms, and let marinate for at least 2 hours in the refrigerator. Serve on top of green salad or as a side. This dish is great on top of Simple Basil Pesto Zucchini Pasta.

Nori Wraps with Tahini Dipping Sauce

Yield: 5 wraps

5 nori sheets

2 avocados, pitted and mashed

1 cup shredded carrots

¼ cup thinly sliced chopped fresh mint

1 cup purple cabbage, shredded

½ cup thinly sliced zucchini

¼ cup raw hemp seeds

Tahini Dipping Sauce

Place nori sheets on a flat work surface. Spread about 1 tablespoon mashed avocado on the bottom quarter edge of each nori sheet. Evenly divide carrots, mint, purple cabbage, zucchini, and raw hemp seeds among nori sheets, and roll. Seal nori sheets by taking a wet paper towel across the inside edges. Serve with Tahini Dipping Sauce.

Simple Basil Pesto Zucchini Pasta

Yield: 2 large bowls

2 large zucchini

Drizzle olive oil

1 carrot, shredded

2 shiitake, crimini, or your favorite mushrooms, sliced

2 TB. Simple Basil Pesto

Pinch sea salt

Pinch freshly ground black pepper

Using a spiralizer or a vegetable peeler, cut zucchini into angel hair–like pasta, and place in a bowl.

Drizzle with a very small amount of olive oil, add carrot and shiitake mushrooms, and toss with Simple Basil Pesto. Season with sea salt and black pepper, and serve.

Variation: This veggie pasta is also fantastic topped with Marinated Portobello Mushrooms or any other variety of fresh veggies you have in the fridge. Try cucumbers, parsnips, broccoli, and yellow squash.

DIY Veggie Pasta

This recipe requires some special equipment to transform your zucchini into angel hair pasta. If you don't have a spiralizer, you can use a vegetable peeler to make ribbonlike pieces with the zucchini.

Vegetable Medley Stir-Fry
Yield: 2 bowls

1 or 2 cloves garlic, minced

1 tsp. fresh minced ginger

1 head broccoli, chopped into bite-size pieces

3 medium carrots, peeled and julienned

1 cup green beans, trimmed

1 cup Chinese snow peas

1 small zucchini, chopped into bite-size pieces

2 celery stalks, chopped into bite-size pieces

½ cup your favorite mushrooms, sliced

1 cup green or red cabbage, shredded

1 head Swiss chard, stems removed, and chopped into bite-size pieces

1 or 2 TB. olive, flaxseed, or hemp seed oil

1 tsp. crushed red pepper flakes (optional)

Handful sprouts (optional)

Fill a large sauté pan with 1 or 2 inches water and set over medium-high heat. Bring water to a boil. Add garlic, ginger, and any particularly hard vegetables like broccoli stems, carrots, green beans, and Chinese snow peas first. Cover, reduce heat to medium-low, and steam for a few minutes, stirring occasionally. Add broccoli crowns, zucchini, celery, mushrooms, and green cabbage and cook, stirring occasionally. Add Swiss chard at the very end, and only cook for 1 or 2 minutes, stirring occasionally. Pour off any excess water, and drink it (or save in a glass jar to use in your next smoothie). Drizzle with olive oil, sprinkle with crushed red pepper flakes (if using) or sprouts (if using), and serve.

Stir-Fry Secrets

This recipe is the foundation of your conscious eating meal plan. You can include whatever nonstarchy vegetables you have in whatever proportions you enjoy. This recipe represents a simple, basic selection of veggies. For more simplicity, just steam one vegetable such as broccoli, zucchini, or green beans. Or go crazy and add whatever you have available. Serve with your favorite nongluten grain or your favorite protein.

If you're preparing a large quantity to save for another meal, remove the vegetables from heat before they're fully cooked and run under cold water. Otherwise, they'll continue cooking and end up softer than you like.

Grain Dishes

Whole grains provide some of the best nutrition available in nature. They are high in enzymes, fiber, vitamins B and E, and they are just the type of carbohydrate your body needs for long-lasting energy. And with nongluten grains, you get all this without the sticky effect of gluten.

The dishes in this chapter are excellent choices for a side dish (remember, just 1 or 2 cups whole grain per meal) alongside your vegetable entrée. You may also want to dive into this section if you're used to heavier, meat-based meals because whole grains can help you feel full and satisfied.

Cooking Great Grains

If you're at all intimidated at the thought of cooking grains from scratch, don't be. It's really quite simple. You just need to know the secrets!

Before you begin, gently rinse your grains so they're free of any dust or residue. Use a handheld colander to hold the measured grains and run them under cold water. Use your hands to gently stir the grains so each gets rinsed.

Next, soak your grains in water for at least 1 hour before cooking. This helps release the phytic acid from the grains, making them easier to digest. To soak, place rinsed grains in a pot and cover with cold, filtered water. Drain and rinse again after soaking and cook with fresh water.

Before cooking, add a pinch of sea salt or a few pieces of sea vegetables (a sprinkle of dulse, sliced nori, or a strip of kombu) to enhance flavor and add nutritional value.

Toasting Grains

Dry-toasting grains allows the grain to cook more evenly, decreases bitterness, and brings out the grains' natural flavor. To dry-toast your grains, pour off the water after soaking and place the grains in a skillet—a cast-iron skillet works great. Set over medium heat, and "toast" the grains for 2 or 3 minutes or until a few start to pop or they smell nutty.

Buckwheat Arame

Yield: 3 cups

¼ cup arame sea vegetables

1 cup raw buckwheat

1⅔ cups water

1 large carrot, shredded

½ white onion, thinly sliced

Drizzle sesame oil

1 scallion, chopped

Place arame sea vegetables in a medium bowl, add water to cover, and soak for at least 5 minutes. Meanwhile, in a medium skillet over medium heat, dry-toast raw buckwheat for 4 or 5 minutes or until nutty and golden brown. In a medium saucepan over high heat, bring 1⅔ cups water to a boil. Slowly add buckwheat, and return to a boil. Reduce heat to medium-low, and simmer for 15 minutes. Remove from heat, and let sit for 15 minutes. Rinse arame, and mix with carrot, white onion, and buckwheat. Drizzle with sesame oil, and sprinkle with fresh scallion before serving.

The Truth About Buckwheat

Buckwheat does not actually contain any wheat, as its name suggests. It's the perfect nongluten grain, except for the fact that it's not really a grain either. Technically, buckwheat is a seed. Nonetheless, it makes an excellent grain alternative. When shopping for buckwheat, look for "raw buckwheat groats." These are raw, a pale green color, and have a mild flavor. "Toasted buckwheat," or kasha, is dark brown with a distinctly earthy taste. All our recipes call for raw buckwheat, which can be toasted or eaten raw after it has been soaked.

Quinoa Watercress Salad

Yield: 4 cups

1 cup quinoa, soaked and rinsed

2 cups water

2 cloves garlic, minced

½ cup chopped scallions

2 TB. chopped fresh mint

2 TB. chopped fresh cilantro

1 cup finely chopped fresh parsley

1 small bunch watercress, chopped

1 cup cucumber, chopped

¼ cup freshly squeezed lemon juice

¼ cup olive oil

½ cup kalamata olives, pitted

Pinch sea salt

Pinch freshly ground black pepper

Crushed red pepper flakes
   (optional)

In a large pot over high heat, combine quinoa and water. Bring to a boil, cover, reduce heat to low, and simmer for 15 to 20 minutes or until all water is absorbed. Remove from heat, and allow quinoa to cool to room temperature. Transfer to a bowl, add garlic and scallions, and mix well. Add mint, cilantro, parsley, watercress, and cucumber, and stir in lemon juice and olive oil. Add kalamata olives, and season with sea salt, black pepper, and crushed red pepper flakes (if using). Set aside for at least 30 minutes before serving to allow flavors to blend.

Savory Brown Rice

Yield: 3 cups

1 TB. sesame oil

1 shallot, chopped

1 cup brown rice, soaked and
   drained

Pinch sea salt

Pinch freshly ground black pepper

2½ cups vegetable stock

1 clove garlic, minced

2 sprigs fresh thyme

1 tsp. dried ground sage

3 green onions, white and green
   parts, thinly sliced

In a medium saucepan over medium heat, warm sesame oil. Add shallot, and sauté for about 3 minutes or until tender. Add brown rice, and stir until coated with oil. Season with sea salt and black pepper. Add vegetable stock, garlic, thyme, and sage. Reduce heat to medium-low, cover, and simmer for about 40 minutes or until water is absorbed. Remove from heat and let stand, covered, for 10 minutes. Remove thyme sprigs, fluff rice with a fork, and toss with green onions before serving.

Simply Millet

Yield: 3½ cups

1 cup millet

6 cups water

2 TB. low-sodium vegetable or chicken broth

1 cup chopped white onion

½ cup chopped fresh parsley

In a large saucepan over high heat, combine millet and water. Bring to a boil, reduce heat to medium-low, and simmer for 15 to 20 minutes or until tender. Drain well and set aside. In a large skillet over medium heat, heat vegetable broth. Add white onion, and cook for 3 or 4 minutes or until onion has softened. Add parsley, and cook for 1 more minute. Stir in cooked millet, toss gently, and serve warm.

Veggie "Fried" Brown Rice

Yield: 4 cups

1 small white onion, chopped

1 TB. sesame oil

2 cloves garlic, minced

1 TB. ginger, minced

1 carrot, diced

1 head broccoli, chopped into bite-size pieces

½ cup frozen peas

2 cups spinach, finely chopped

3 scallions, chopped

4 cups cooked brown rice

2 TB. Ume plum vinegar

½ tsp. crushed red pepper flakes

In a wok or large skillet over medium-high heat, sauté white onion in sesame oil for about 5 minutes. Add garlic, and cook, stirring frequently, for 2 more minutes. Add ginger, carrot, broccoli, and peas, and cook, stirring frequently, for a few more minutes or until carrots and broccoli start to soften. Add spinach, scallions, and cooked brown rice, and mix well. Pour in Ume plum vinegar, and continue to stir for 1 minute. Serve warm, topping with crushed red pepper flakes.

Wild Rice Salad

Yield: 3 cups

3 cloves garlic, minced

1½ TB. Dijon mustard

½ tsp. plus 1 pinch sea salt

½ tsp. freshly ground black pepper

3 drops liquid stevia, or 1 tsp. honey

½ cup rice wine vinegar

1 cup uncooked wild rice, soaked and rinsed

3 cups water

½ cup freshly squeezed lemon juice

3 scallions (including tops), sliced

1 head Swiss chard, de-stemmed and shredded

½ cup white button, shiitake, crimini, or your favorite mushrooms, sliced

In a glass jar with a lid, combine garlic, Dijon mustard, ½ teaspoon sea salt, black pepper, stevia, and rice wine vinegar. Shake well, and set aside. In a large pot over high heat, combine rice and water and remaining pinch sea salt. Bring to a boil, reduce heat to low, cover, and simmer for 45 to 50 minutes or until all water is absorbed. In a medium bowl, toss warm wild rice with lemon juice. Add scallions, Swiss chard, and mushrooms, and toss with dressing. Season with additional sea salt and black pepper, cover, and refrigerate for 2 to 4 hours before serving.

Meat Dishes

As we've promised throughout the book, meat lovers do not need to feel deprived during the Conscious Cleanse. In this chapter, you'll see that we like to broil or bake, rather than fry, most meat dishes. Using these techniques requires less oil and doesn't char your meat. If you were raised on "hockey puck" hamburgers, consider cooking your meat more moderately for a couple weeks.

Practice shifting your perspective a little and thinking of your meat dish as a side dish to your delicious plate of raw or lightly steamed veggies!

Baked Cod with Lemon and Olive Oil

Yield: 4 cod fillets

4 (4- to 6-oz.) cod fillets

1½ TB. freshly squeezed lemon juice

1 TB. olive oil

2 cloves garlic, minced

½ tsp. dried thyme

Pinch sea salt

Pinch freshly ground black pepper

¼ tsp. paprika (optional)

Preheat the oven to 400°F. Arrange cod fillets in a 13×9-inch baking dish. Drizzle with lemon juice and olive oil; sprinkle with garlic, thyme, sea salt, black pepper, and paprika (if using); and lightly rub in spices. Bake for 15 to 20 minutes or until cod flesh is completely opaque but still juicy.

Variation: Serve with the pan juices drizzled over the top and alongside steamed veggies.

Basic Baked Chicken Breasts

Yield: 4 chicken breasts

1 TB. olive oil

1 clove garlic, minced

4 medium boneless and skinless chicken breast halves

Pinch sea salt

Pinch freshly ground black pepper

1 TB. fresh oregano, minced

1 TB. fresh rosemary, minced

1 TB. fresh spearmint, minced

Preheat the oven to 450°F. Line a baking pan with aluminum foil. In a small bowl, combine olive oil and garlic. Brush both sides of each chicken breast half with olive oil–garlic mixture, and sprinkle each side with sea salt, black pepper, oregano, rosemary, and spearmint. Place chicken in the prepared baking pan, and bake for 8 to 10 minutes. Flip over chicken, and bake for 8 to 10 more minutes or until juices run clear.

Variation: If you don't have the fresh herbs, you can use dried spices instead. Also, get creative with what you've already got! Experiment with different combinations of spices.

Fresh Versus Dried Herbs

Fresh herbs tend to have a more robust flavor, but dried herbs are a great alternative when fresh aren't available. The general guideline is to use three times more fresh herbs than dried herbs in a recipe. For example, use 1 tablespoon dried herbs or 3 tablespoons fresh herbs. But don't get too hung up on the math. Just know you'll use more fresh herbs than dried in your preparations and you'll be fine!

Broiled Lamb Chops

Yield: 4 lamb chops

4 lamb chops

Pinch sea salt

Pinch freshly ground black pepper

1 clove garlic

4 lemon wedges

Preheat the broiler to medium. Sprinkle lamb chops with sea salt and black pepper. Cut garlic clove in $\frac{1}{2}$ and rub over lamb chops. Place chops in a baking pan, and broil 3 or 4 inches from the heat source for 2 or 3 minutes per side or until nicely browned on both sides. Watch not to overcook. Serve with lemon wedges.

Make It Medium

Some broilers have low, medium, and high settings, but others only have a single broiler setting. If you have the option, start with a medium setting to avoid charring.

Ginger Broiled Salmon
Yield: 2 salmon fillets

1 TB. sesame oil

¼ cup water

2 tsp. minced ginger

1 TB. Ume plum or apple cider vinegar

2 (4-oz.) wild salmon fillets

In a small bowl, combine sesame oil, water, ginger, and Ume plum vinegar. Place wild salmon fillets skin side down in a shallow baking dish, cover with marinade, and refrigerate for 30 minutes. Preheat the broiler to medium. Remove salmon from the refrigerator, and broil skin side down 3 or 4 inches from the heat source for 6 to 8 minutes. Baste with remaining marinade once or twice while broiling. Use any remaining baking pan juices as a sauce, and serve alongside steamed veggies or with a salad.

Lemon Pepper Chicken
Yield: 4 chicken breasts

4 boneless, skinless chicken breasts

Pinch freshly ground black pepper

Pinch sea salt

Zest of 2 lemons

Juice of 2 lemons

4 TB. extra-virgin olive oil

Coat chicken breasts with black pepper, and season lightly with sea salt. In a small bowl, combine lemon zest and lemon juice with extra-virgin olive oil. Place a large skillet over medium-high heat, and fill the pan with ¼ inch marinade. Add chicken breasts, and cook for 6 or 7 minutes per side or until no longer pink, adding more marinade as needed to keep chicken lightly covered while cooking. Transfer chicken to a serving platter, and brush with remaining pan juices.

Red Ruby Trout Salad

Yield: 3 or 4 cups

1 lb. rainbow trout fillets, with skin

½ tsp. sea salt

1 tsp. freshly ground black pepper

2 TB. olive oil, plus more for garnish

½ cup freshly squeezed lemon juice

2 stalks celery, chopped

½ cup red onion, chopped

½ TB. fresh tarragon, finely chopped

4 cups mixed field greens

1 lemon wedge

Preheat an ovenproof skillet (cast iron is perfect) over medium-high heat for 3 or 4 minutes. Preheat the broiler to medium, and move the oven rack 4 inches from the heat source. Place rainbow trout fillets skin side down in the hot skillet.

Sprinkle with ¼ teaspoon sea salt and ½ teaspoon black pepper, and cook for 6 minutes or until flesh turns opaque halfway up fillet. Place the hot skillet under the broiler, and cook for a few minutes until top browns. Remove from the broiler, peel away burned skin, and allow to cool. Tear cooled trout apart into bite-size pieces, and place in a bowl. Add olive oil, lemon juice, celery, red onion, tarragon, remaining ¼ teaspoon sea salt, and remaining ½ teaspoon black pepper, and toss to coat. Serve over a bed of mixed field greens, garnished with lemon wedge, and a drizzle of olive oil.

Variation: For a quicker alternative, substitute 2 (6-ounce) cans wild salmon in water for the trout fillets.

Terrific Trout

This quick and easy recipe uses the trout's skin to cook the fish. Be sure you have the exhaust fan on for the smoke!

Turkey Lettuce Wraps

Yield: 12 wraps with ½ to 1 cup filling per wrap

2 TB. sesame oil

2 cloves garlic, minced

1½ lb. ground turkey

5 or 6 green onions, cut 2 in. past
  white part, and chopped

1 cup carrots, chopped

1 cup shiitake mushrooms, chopped

1 cup celery, chopped

2 TB. minced ginger

¼ tsp. crushed red pepper flakes

1 cup fresh whole cilantro leaves

Pinch sea salt

Pinch freshly ground black pepper

1 TB. honey (optional)

1 head napa cabbage or romaine or
  Bibb lettuce

In a large skillet or wok over medium heat, heat sesame oil and garlic for 2 minutes. Add ground turkey, stirring to break larger chunks into small pieces, and cook for 6 to 8 minutes or until turkey is crumbly and no longer pink. Stir in green onions, carrots, shiitake mushrooms, celery, ginger, and crushed red pepper flakes, and cook for 5 minutes. Vegetables should be lightly cooked, not wilted. Add cilantro leaves, and cook for a few more minutes. Remove skillet from heat, and season with sea salt and black pepper. For a dash of sweetness, add honey (if using), and cook for 2 minutes. Spoon ½ to 1 cup filling onto 1 napa cabbage leaf, roll or fold in half, and serve.

Variation: For more heat, add another ¼ teaspoon crushed red pepper flakes.

Turkey Spinach Burgers

Yield: 4 burgers

1 lb. ground turkey breast

1¼ cups spinach, chopped

½ cup red onion, chopped

½ cup sesame seeds

3 TB. minced ginger

2 TB. olive or sesame oil

Pinch sea salt

Pinch freshly ground black pepper

Preheat the oven to 375°F. Line a baking pan with aluminum foil. In a large bowl, use your hands to combine turkey breast, spinach, red onion, sesame seeds, ginger, olive oil, sea salt, and black pepper. Form mixture into 4 (4-ounce) patties, and place on the prepared baking pan. Bake for 30 minutes, turning once.

Wild West Buffalo

Yield: 2 steaks

2 TB. olive oil

2 TB. balsamic vinegar

2 TB. fresh rosemary, chopped

2 TB. fresh thyme, chopped

4 cloves garlic, minced

Zest of 1 lemon

2 bison steaks

In a medium bowl, whisk together olive oil, balsamic vinegar, rosemary, thyme, garlic, and lemon zest. Add bison steaks, and marinate in the refrigerator for 2 hours or overnight. Preheat the broiler to medium. Drain bison steaks from marinade, and pat dry. (Excess marinade will burn.) Place bison steaks on a broiler pan, and broil 4 or 5 inches from heat source for 4 or 5 minutes per side. Adjust cook time for thickness of steaks.

Variation: If you don't have a broiler or broiling pan, you can cook your bison in a large cast-iron skillet. Preheat the oven to 500°F while you also preheat the skillet over medium-high heat until it's smoking. Sprinkle sea salt on the skillet. Add bison steaks, and immediately transfer the skillet to the bottom oven rack. Cook for 4 or 5 minutes per side or until fully cooked.

Thin Is In

When cooking with bison steaks, thinner cuts of meat are best. Try to use pieces less than 1 inch thick.

Sweet Alternatives

Yes, we have a sweet tooth, too! It's great to add a sweet treat occasionally—especially during transition days—but notice if you're always grabbing for the sweet stuff. Giving yourself a break helps reduce your cravings and benefits your long-term health goals.

In this chapter, we share some sweet cleanse-friendly recipes, as well as a few to save for after your cleanse.

Banana Chips
Yield: about 60 chips

4 bananas, peeled
¼ cup freshly squeezed lemon juice

Preheat the oven to 200°F. Cut bananas in ¼-inch discs, and sprinkle or lightly brush with lemon juice. Place banana discs on a parchment paper–lined baking sheet, and bake for 2 or 3 hours, or longer for a crispier consistency. Remove chips from the oven and cool on the baking sheet to harden even more.

Variation: For a sweeter treat, sprinkle with ground cinnamon!

Frozen Fruit Bites
Yield: 4 cups

2 cups grapes
1 medium cantaloupe, peeled and cubed (2 cups)

Place grapes and cantaloupe cubes in a freezer bag, and freeze until solid. Enjoy straight from the freezer. Kids love these!

Variation: Any other fruits, cut into bite-size pieces, also work in this recipe.

Mint Madness*

Yield: 2 cups

This recipe is for transition days and after your cleanse only.

1 cup Homemade Almond Milk

1 banana, peeled (frozen for creamy texture)

2 TB. raw cacao powder

1½ TB. raw cacao nibs

1 tsp. maca powder

10 fresh mint leaves, or to taste

3 or 4 ice cubes

In a high-speed blender, combine Homemade Almond Milk, banana, raw cacao powder, raw cacao nibs, maca powder, mint leaves, and ice cubes until smooth. Serve immediately.

Raw Blueberry Pie

Yield: 1 pie

1 cup raw walnuts

½ cup dates, pitted

1 tsp. vanilla extract

½ tsp. ground cinnamon

Pinch sea salt

4 cups organic fresh blueberries

1 TB. honey

In a food processor fitted with an S blade, combine raw walnuts,

dates, vanilla extract, cinnamon, and sea salt until smooth. Press mixture evenly into a pie dish, and refrigerate for about 1 hour or until crust is hard. Meanwhile, in the food processor fitted with an S blade, combine blueberries and honey. Pour into chilled crust, and refrigerate for at least 2 hours before serving.

Raw Brownies*

Yield: 20 small brownies

This recipe is for transition days and after your cleanse only.

1 cup raw walnuts

1 cup dates, pitted

¼ cup raw cacao powder

In a high-speed blender, combine raw walnuts and dates until smooth. Add raw cacao powder and blend again. Press mixture into an

8×8-inch baking dish lined with wax paper. Refrigerate for at least 30 minutes before serving.

Variation: For more chocolaty decadence, add another ¼ cup raw cacao powder.

Quick, Easy, Delicious

This is our go-to potluck dessert! It's always a crowd-pleaser—
if the brownies last long enough to make it out of the house,
that is.

Sweet Herbal Popsicles
Yield: 16 to 20 popsicles

2 cups brewed hibiscus,
   peppermint, or cinnamon herbal
   tea, cooled to room temperature
2 TB. freshly squeezed lime or
   lemon juice
Stevia or honey (optional)

In a pitcher, combine herbal tea,
lime juice, and stevia (if using).
Pour mixture into ice-cube trays
(or Popsicle molds). To secure
toothpicks, cover ice-cube trays
with plastic wrap, poke toothpicks
through plastic, and freeze.

Index

C

H

I